Mental Handicap

Mental Handicap

Edited by

Alan Parrish

with the assistance of

Alison Morton-Cooper

and with contributions from

Anthony R. Thompson
Karen Morgan
Amanda Gunner
Gillian James
Mary Birchenall
Pat Brudenell
Tom Keighley
Peter Birchenall

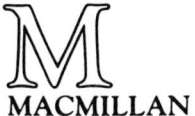

MACMILLAN

First published 1987

Published by
MACMILLAN EDUCATION LTD
Houndmills, Basingstoke, Hampshire RG21 2XS
and London
Companies and representatives
throughout the world

Printed in Great Britain by
Scotprint Ltd,
Musselburgh, Scotland

British Library Cataloguing in Publication Data
Mental handicap. — (The Essentials of nursing).
1. Psychiatric nursing
I. Parrish, Alan   II. Morton-Cooper,
Alison   III. Series
610.73′68   RC440
ISBN 0–333–44467–1

The contributors

Mary Birchenall, RNMH, BA.

Peter Birchenall, RNMH, RGN, DipN(Lond), RNT, MA.

Pat Brudenell, RMN, RDTh, DipTh, AIST, CertEd, formerly worked for over seven years in the further education sector with students with special needs. Freelance dramatherapist. Author of *The Other Side of Profound Handicap* (Macmillan Education, 1986).

Amanda Gunner, RNMH, DipN(Lond), CertEd, RNT, is currently working for the Royal College of Nursing as Student Association Officer for the Association of Nursing Students.

Gillian James, RNMH, RGN, RCNT, FEdTCert, is currently Clinical Teacher at the Warwickshire School of Nursing, and was formerly a ward sister who has worked in Derbyshire, Cheshire, Buckinghamshire and Warwickshire.

Tom Keighley, RGN, RMN, NDNCert, RCNT, DipN, BA, is currently Director of Nursing with the Waltham Forest Health Authority.

Karen Morgan, RNMH, is currently studying for the RGN at King's College Hospital, London.

Alison Morton-Cooper, RGN, trained as a newspaper and periodical journalist with the *Dundee Courier* Group in Dundee, and after extensive voluntary work in mental handicap and psychiatric hospitals, trained in general nursing at St Mary's Hospital, Paddington, qualifying in 1982.

Anthony R. Thompson, RNMH, RMN, DipN(Lond), CertEd, RNT, BEd, is currently Education Officer (Mental Handicap) with the English National Board for Nursing, Midwifery and Health Visiting.

Contents

Foreword to the series

This series of textbooks offers a fresh approach to the study of nursing. The aim is to give those beginning a career in nursing, and those already qualified, opportunities for reflection to broaden their approach to nursing education and to identify their own nursing values. The text includes material currently required by those preparing for qualification as a nurse and offers a basis for developing knowledge by individual studies. It should also assist qualified nurses returning to nursing, and those wishing to gain further insight into the nursing curriculum.

The authors of each book in the series are from widely differing nursing backgrounds, and, as experienced teachers of nursing or midwifery, they are well aware of the difficulties faced by nursing students searching for meaning from a mass of factual information. The nurse has to practise in the real world, and in reality nursing students need to learn to practise with confidence and understanding. The authors have therefore collaborated to illustrate this new perspective by making full use of individual nursing care plans to present the knowledge required by the nursing student in the most appropriate and relevant way. These textbooks can therefore be used in a wide variety of nursing programmes.

The practice of nursing—as a profession and as a career—and the education of the nurse to fulfil her role are both affected by national and international trends. The Nurses, Midwives and Health Visitors Act 1979 in the United Kingdom, the Treaty of Rome and the European Community nursing directives 1977, as well as the deliberations and publications of the International Council of Nurses and the World Health Organization, all make an impact upon the preparation and the practice of the nurse throughout the world.

Nursing values may not have changed over the past one hundred years, but society and the patterns of both life and care have changed, and are constantly changing. It is particularly important, therefore, to restate the essentials of nursing in the light of current practice and future trends.

Throughout this series the focus is on nursing and on the individual—the person requiring care and the person giving care—and emphasises the need for continuity between home and hospital care. *Neighbourhood Nursing—A Focus for Care*, the Report of the Community Nursing Review under the chairmanship of Julia Cumberlege (HMSO, 1986) has drawn attention to this need. The developing role of the nurse in primary care and in health education is reflected throughout this series. The authors place their emphasis on the whole person, and nursing care studies and care plans are used to promote understanding of the clinical, social, psychological and spiritual aspects of care for the individual.

Each book introduces the various aspects of the curriculum for general nursing: the special needs of (1) those requiring acute care; (2) the elderly; (3) children; (4) the mentally ill; and (5) the mentally handicapped. The last is a new text in The Essentials of Nursing—edited by a well-known and respected nurse for the mentally handicapped and with contributors experienced in differing aspects of caring for people with mental handicap. The text on maternity and neonatal care, written by a midwifery teacher, provides the material for nursing students and would be helpful to those undertaking preparation for further health visiting education.

The authors wish to acknowledge their gratitude for the assistance they have received from members of the Editorial Board, and from all those who have contributed to their work—patients and their relatives, students, qualified nurses and colleagues—too numerous to mention by name. To all those nurse teachers who have read some of the texts, offering constructive criticism and comment from their special knowledge, we offer our grateful thanks.

1987   Sheila Collins

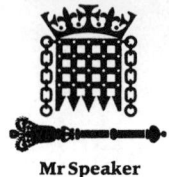

Speaker's House   Westminster   London   SW1A 0AA

Foreword

Mental handicap is a central issue in health care provision for today and tomorrow. For over 20 years I have been President of the Croydon Branch of the Royal Society for Mentally Handicapped Children and Adults and I have taken a close interest in St Lawrence's Hospital, Caterham. It is particularly rewarding, therefore, to be associated with a team responsible for developing this text in The Essentials of Nursing series. The hallmark of all those involved with this book—Sheila Collins, Alan Parrish and the contributors—is their genuine and professional commitment to improving the standard of care and provision for mentally handicapped people. The content of this book emphasises that the mentally handicapped person is an individual with his own rights, and needs to be given an opportunity to live as an integral member of his local community. It is a positive book, about facing and solving problems practically and cheerfully.

I warmly recommend the book to students, nurses, teachers, parents and all those whose life and work brings them in close contact with mentally handicapped people. I hope that all of you will be enriched by the themes and ideas developed.

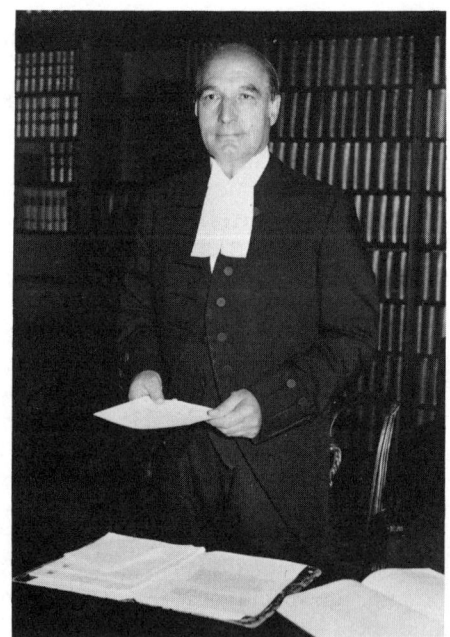

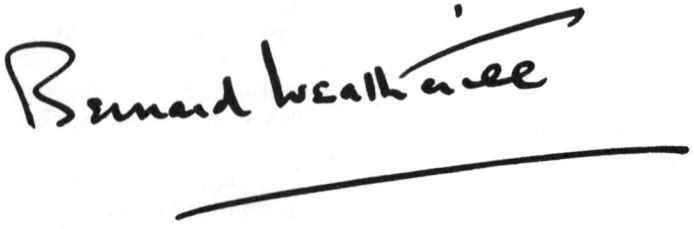

Preface

This book is designed to offer to readers an introduction to mental handicap nursing. It has been added to the six books in The Essentials of Nursing series, to focus on particular issues which arise in this specialised form of nursing.

Mental handicap nursing is about helping people with a mental handicap and their relatives to experience a normal way of life—enjoying the things we so often take for granted. The nurse encourages the person to learn, and while providing care, promotes an environment in which the values, customs and spiritual beliefs of the individual are respected in a rapidly changing society. Such nursing is based on the recognition that each person has a right to make choices, and to be involved in activities which help **him** to develop **his** full potential.

The work is demanding, and calls for special aptitude, for patience, for an understanding that each person is unique, and for co-operation between a wide variety of people from different professional backgrounds whose aim is to educate and help people with mental handicap. Skills based on knowledge and an awareness of the complexity of the issues which arise in such teamwork are essential—and are acquired by learning from the experience in a supportive and caring setting.

This text is intended for those following a course of preparation for registration as a nurse for the mentally handicapped, to be used in conjunction with the other books in the series: in particular, *Essentials of Nursing—An Introduction, Care of the Child* and *Care of the Elderly*. It may also assist nurses already qualified or those returning to practise in this form of caring. At this time, when the nurse's role is extending, when the emphasis is on care in the community and in residential settings, and when expectations of a fully comprehensive service for mentally handicapped people have yet to be realised, it is vital that the nurse be fully aware of the sources of help and the resources needed to meet the challenges and uncertainties of the future.

Throughout the series the aim is to clarify the differences between disability, handicap and disease, and to identify the role of the nurse, in health education and in promoting health.

This book, an addition to the series, draws together the collective thoughts of eight experienced nurses each of whom strongly believes in the need to share their knowledge and skills, to foster and maintain the contribution the nurse makes to this special service to humanity.

London W1, 1987   A.P.

Acknowledgements

The editor and authors would like to thank Miss S. Collins, OBE, BA, RGN, RSCN, RNT, FRCN, for her guidance and advice during the preparation of this book.

The cover photograph was taken by Ed Barber for *Nursing Times*.

A note on the series style

Throughout this book, in keeping with the other titles in this series, the term *nursing student* has been used to mean *both* student or pupil nurses *and* trained nurses who are undertaking post-basic training or who are keeping up to date with the recent literature. For clarity and consistency throughout the series the nurse is described as *she*; this is done without prejudice to men who are nurses or nursing students. Similarly, the patient is sometimes referred to as *he*, when the gender is not specifically mentioned.

Care plans, which are used throughout the books in this series, are indicated by a coloured corner flash to distinguish them from the rest of the text.

Chapter 1

Introduction: Nurse education and mental handicap care

by Anthony R. Thompson

The person who undertakes to train as a competent mental handicap nurse during this decade will have to be capable of making many adjustments. She will be expected to question her own life's philosophy together with the principles which underpin the concepts of contemporary care provision for a person with a mental handicap.

Those responsible for the vocational preparation of the nurse have to be increasingly aware of the importance of giving the nursing student access to the knowledge and experiences which will result in a highly skilled and competent practitioner.

Mental handicap nursing is no longer synonymous with hospital-based care, and the student will have this point reinforced many times during professional education. Nursing in general has entered a transitional phase but mental handicap nursing in particular is increasingly seen as undergoing both a conceptual and an 'image' change.

The education of the nurse has followed the needs of the service delivery, and until the flexibility of the 1982 syllabus (English National Board for Nursing, Midwifery and Health Visiting, 1982) was incorporated into the local curriculum, the traditional and stereotyped image of the nurse was perpetuated. Such an education relied heavily on a physiological science basis of knowledge. The new syllabus seeks to alter this state and thus to portray a more relevant, accurate and appropriate model of mental handicap nursing. The need for such a change was recognised by the Chief Nursing Officer at the Department of Health and Social Security in her letter to senior members of the nursing profession (DHSS CNO (85) 5). These and related issues have also been addressed in two relevant units of work by the English National Board for Nursing, Midwifery and Health Visiting (1985a, b). I believe one of the major difficulties still encountered by the nursing student is coming to terms with such a legacy, together with future attempts to bridge the gap between the models and educational ideals of the 1970s and 1980s and the sometimes harsh reality of care provision in restricted environments. These difficulties present a great challenge to curriculum planners and require a lot of effort and mutual support. Sound guidance, supervision of practice and skilled monitoring are implicit within the new syllabus.

The philosophy

In common with other systems of education, the design of the syllabus promotes the vocational preparation of the nurse as a worth-while activity. In the heart of a system of education can be found the ideals and values it sets out to attain. Such ideals are determined by beliefs, and the 1982 syllabus is constructed around a belief which recognises and accepts that a person with a mental handicap has the same human value as any other member of society. The principles and ideals are now reflected in the planned teaching programmes. This is a necessary condition, because if the beliefs and ideals are to be firmly established in the care setting, then a system of education must logically follow in order to perpetuate them.

(a) The evolution of the philosophy

The previous decade has seen rapid and complex developments in organised care for the handicapped person. Many of these developments contributed directly to the syllabus design. It has been constructed to reflect significant advances in knowledge and care skills together with a refinement of attitudes towards the handicapped person in society. It does this while retaining elements of accountable practice which form the integrity of the nursing profession as a whole.

The nursing student will be prepared to meet the demands which are implicit within the syllabus philosophy and should be expected to fulfil the following role:

The function of the nurse for people with a mental handicap is directly and skilfully to assist the individual and his family, whatever the handicap, in the acquisition, development and maintenance of those skills that, given the necessary ability, could be performed unaided: and to do this in such a way as to enable independence to be gained as rapidly and fully as possible, in an environment that maintains a quality of life that would be acceptable to fellow citizens of the same age. (Adapted from Henderson (1966))

Mental handicap nursing—a skill-based activity

The course teacher and the nursing student enter into a moral contract which desires that learning and teaching is implemented within the framework of:

1. The principles of the syllabus.
2. The definition of a nurse for people with a mental handicap.

In order to achieve this, it has to be recognised that providing nursing care for the person who has a mental handicap is a highly skilled activity. The foundation for such skills is to be found in a rational and systematic approach to nursing care. This approach uses a problem-solving method to determine the needs of people with a mental handicap and others involved in care provision. The skills that will be required in order to achieve competency will be not only the traditionally taught 'hard' skills of a procedural nature, but also what Spencer (1979) has called 'soft skills'.

Among the more important of soft skills to be learned (and they can only be taught in an appropriate environment) are Non-Verbal or Accurate Empathy. This is really the ability to actually 'hear' what a person is 'really' saying or meaning in a negotiation.

The other skill is that of Positive Expectation, or what Rosenthal and Jacobson (1968) call the Pygmalion effect. This is a strong belief in the underlying dignity and worth of others different from oneself—and the ability to maintain this under stress. A nurse can learn such skills and will continue throughout her career to improve her performance. Interestingly, these skills are not dependent on racial, sexual or socio-economic status. This is of value when both the student and the teacher consider the wide background of their peers and the diverse cultures of people who have a handicap.

Towards competency

The Nurses, Midwives and Health Visitors Act 1979 requires all nurses to be competent. One of the effects of achieving the competencies will be to bring the nursing student into greater contact with other professionals and informal carers. In the process of becoming competent, the nurse will have strengthened the partnership bond within which the process of nursing must exist.

It is possible to show diagramatically how the planners of the 1982 curriculum, the course leaders and the students match the needs of service provision with the educational needs of the practitioner.

The nursing student may have to face various reactions to change quite early in training. A major reason for this is that the changing principles and philosophy which influence service delivery and education, demand new skills and an alteration in attitude towards the role.

A well-planned total learning environment should assist the nursing student to acquire the body of knowledge which reflects the whole process of nursing the person with a mental handicap. In order to facilitate this for the student, the course planners should strive to design a curriculum that promotes educational progression. Progress through the training period may be seen in:

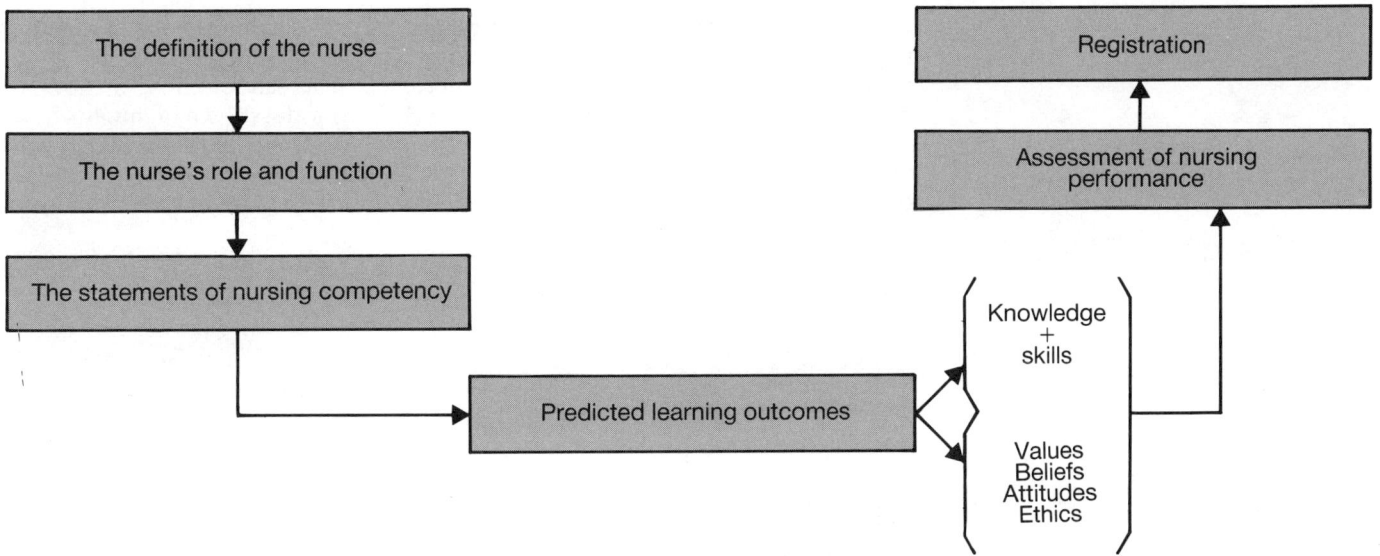

Figure 1.1 *A specification of mental handicap nursing competence*

1. *Variety of learning experience*—here the nursing student is not expected to repeat learning experiences unless there is a planned purpose and aim.
2. *Matching*—the design of the course should aim to link the teaching of mental handicap nursing skills with the learning style of the nursing student.
3. *Sequencing*—the planned learning environment should enable the nursing student to extend and build upon previous vocational and life experience.

The demands that a competency-based curriculum makes on course tutors is that they have to be sensitive to individual learning needs rather than offer instruction. The demand on the nursing student is that she has to be willing to be an independent and critical thinker.

The learning experience

Although the 1982 syllabus is divided into some nineteen sections, these sections are not to be considered as discrete areas of knowledge. This point is of equal importance to both tutor and student. The tutor plans teaching which promotes the integration of the nine 'core' sections which are considered to be valid areas of knowledge, skills and attitudes, together with the ten sections which represent areas of practical common experience. The nursing student needs to apply her acquired knowledge of the core concepts throughout the training period, and to adapt them in a variety of settings.

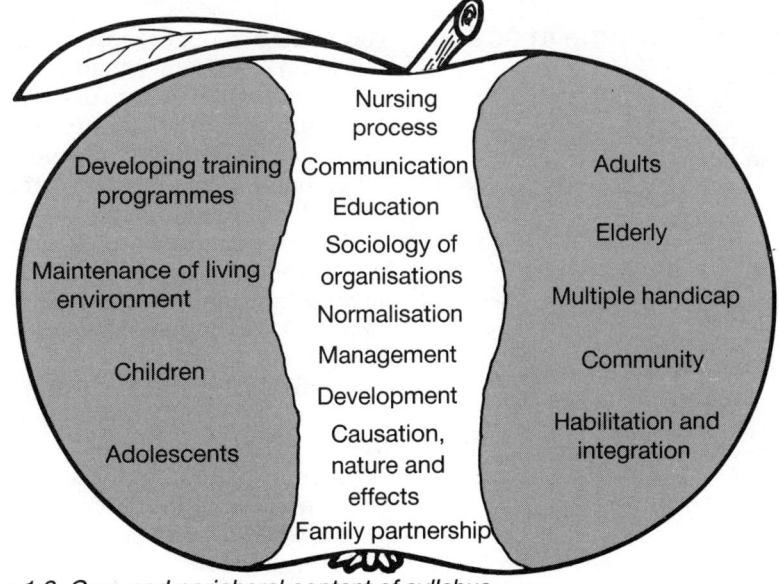

Figure 1.2 *Core and peripheral content of syllabus*

The following example is just one typical way in which a school of nursing might plan a 146 week learning experience. The curriculum has been designed using modules or units of learning experience. The school chose a rational curriculum model as illustrated in Figure 1.3. The model shown highlights how each part of the curriculum interacts with another. The evaluation aspect will allow for changes to occur as a result of such things as an increase in the choice of placements, new residential settings, alteration of teaching styles as tutors change, and so on.

In order to implement this model, it is likely that the nursing student would follow the type of planned, allocated experience seen in Figure 1.4.

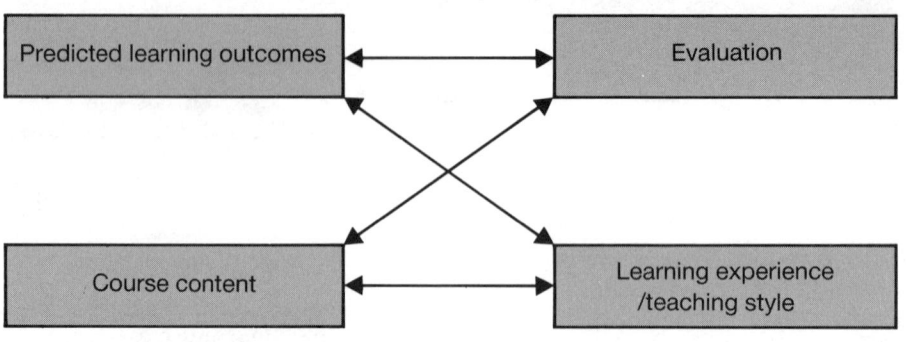

Figure 1.3 A curriculum model

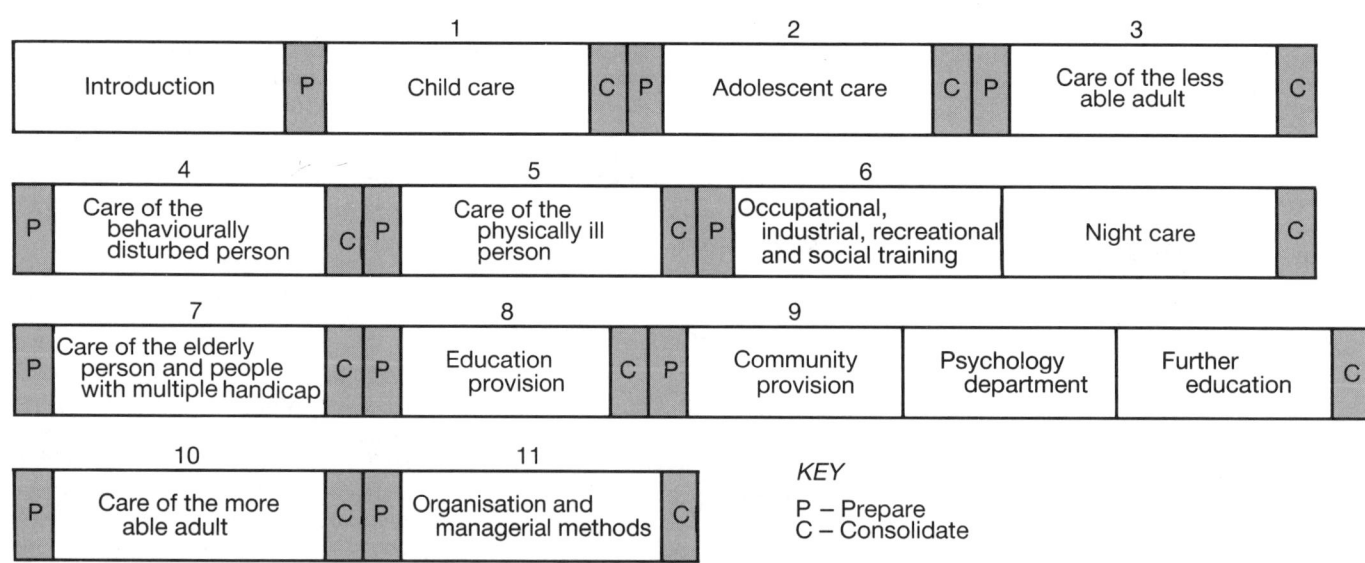

Figure 1.4 A planned allocation for the learning experience

(a) The programme in action

The nursing student following this programme will have been introduced to the developmental sequence of forthcoming experiences.

Typically, the majority of the experience in **module 1** will be found outside of the health service. The tutors have organised normal childhood development and the organisation of a healthy living environment.

In **module 2** the experience of caring for adolescents is one that can often be easily identified with by the majority of nursing students. The tutor can 'cash in' on the students' previous experience of life. The student acquires good insight into the additional problems the handicapped person has in growing up in an increasingly complex society. Relationships and marriage are issues likely to be identified for discussion when tutors and students consolidate this unit of experience.

In **module 3** the nursing student may find that much of the experience will take place in the hospital setting. Techniques of behavioural analysis and the study of handicapping clinical conditions will be covered in this module. During this placement the student will have the opportunity to gain increased understanding of the discomfort and isolation that may be experienced by a person who has a severe disability.

During **module 4** the nursing student will gain experience in the special aspects of care and management of people who may exhibit behavioural disturbance. Such disturbance may result in aggressive or antisocial practices, and careful monitoring of this placement will be needed. This experience is often viewed as most valuable by the student as the professional knowledge, skills and attitudes being developed will be utilised to the full.

The nature of the health service provision for sick people means that they are often returned to their home quite quickly after a period of hospital treatment. This phenomenon occurs with disabled people, too, and the nursing student who gains experience in general nursing care in **module 5** can feel able to offer a better service in the variety of settings in which people with a mental handicap live. Of particular importance is the ability to deal with first-aid emergencies and the more specialised care of people who have gross orthopaedic handicapping conditions.

Aspects of occupational/industrial/recreational and social training will be experienced by various methods in **module 6**. A nursing student may find this experience condensed into a placement in one specialist unit or have the opportunity to have short placements in various settings. It is here that insight into the nature of interdisciplinary care can be gained and a recognition of the need for 'life-skills' to be taught to people with a mental handicap.

It is a fact that a significant number of people who have a mental handicap are over the normal retirement age. A proportion of these people have an associated physical disability or psychiatric disorder. In **module 7** the nursing student will learn the complexity of skills required to offer effective care, and gain experience in such areas as motor skill development, and appreciation of specific sensory, emotional and perceptual difficulties.

An extension of the experience gained in the care of children is likely during **module 8**. The nursing student might find herself attached to one local authority school for children with learning difficulties. Alternatively, she may spend time in more than one establishment, including an ordinary primary or secondary school. The basics of teaching methodology will be learned and the opportunity can be taken to apply these methods in other than formal educational settings.

It is during this type of allocation that the student begins to realise the need for continued education to be made available for the person with a mental handicap. Experience in further and adult education may be gained but is usually dependent upon the local provision of such a service.

In **module 9** the experience of specialist community provision is usually one of the most enjoyable for the course tutor and the nursing student. Although a complex allocation, both the theory and practical elements are intense. Increasingly, the student may find her experience monitored by a practice supervisor who has a wide experience of community services. Among the areas likely to be experienced will be the provision of local services, local attitudes towards maintaining or integrating people with a mental handicap into society, the implication of political decisions, evaluation of proposed services and a comparison of standards of care, together with the quality of life for relatives and non-professional carers.

During **module 10** the nursing student will be able to gain first-hand knowledge of the practical difficulties that a more able person with a mental handicap may have to overcome. Among these will be issues concerning limitations of choice and sexual expression. It is during this type of placement that the student is likely to realise that it is not necessarily the traditional hospital which offers a restricted environment. The course tutor may find that this allocation allows work to be undertaken which reinforces the need for a more positive social image for the person with a handicap, together with a more informed professional image of the nurse.

It can be anticipated that during **module 11**, the latter phase of training, the learner will look to her teachers, to prepare her for an increased level of responsibility. This will mean enhancing organisational skills and increasing the ability to plan and handle change. Negotiating and working with professional colleagues takes on a greater significance, and decision-making and leadership roles may emerge.

It must be stated that whatever the planned experience and whatever the aims of the course, each nursing student as an individual will contribute and take from the environment accordingly. Not only are these factors recognised in the 1982 syllabus; they should be taken into account when the student undergoes periodic assessment of her professional capabilities. If this aspect is ignored by either the students or their teachers, then there will be a tendency to fail to recognise students' particular strengths and weaknesses, not only during the training period, but also in their future professional development.

(b) The process and the product

Whatever the perspectives of the syllabus planners, only the wise craftsmanship of the local curriculum designers can ensure that it matches the reality of the expectations of the course. It is a positive sign that an increasing number of nursing students sit as equal partners on the curriculum-planning group. The curriculum that is produced will be influenced by many factors, including a sound knowledge base. This base includes a high value being placed on knowledge of nursing practice, as well as the more formal bodies of knowledge.

It can be seen from Figure 1.5 that this is a process which recognises experience of nursing practice as a major contribution. It is this aspect that will give credibility and allow the nurse trained within the framework of this syllabus to make a worth-while contribution to the care of the person with a mental handicap.

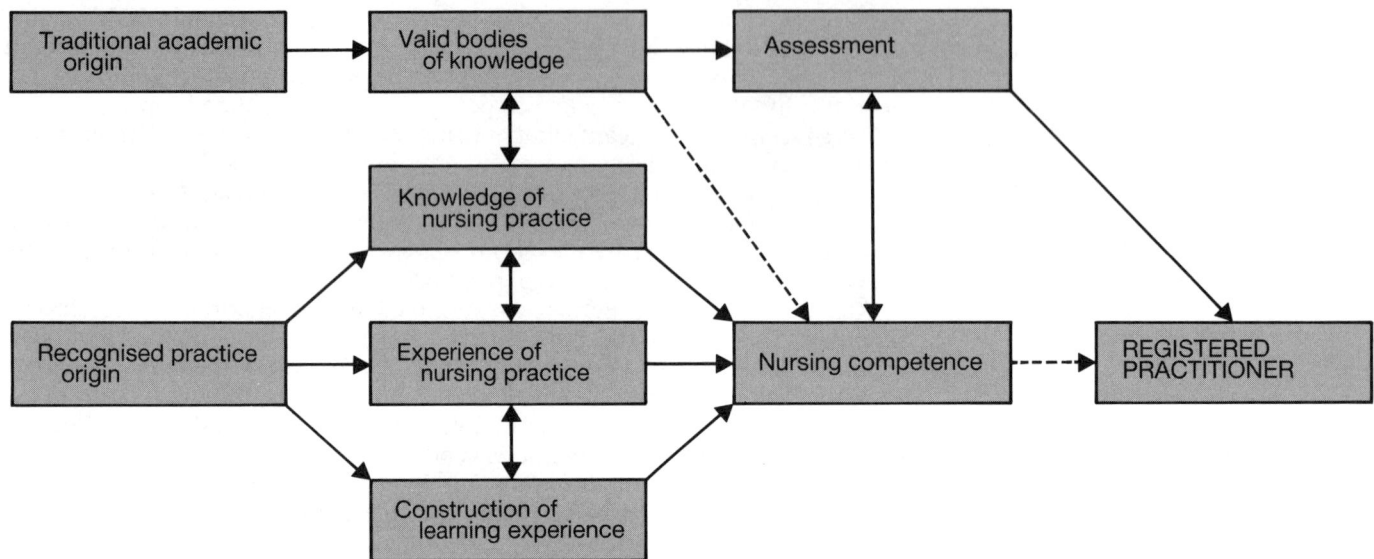

Figure 1.5 Origins and outcomes of mental handicap nursing

Close examination of this process reveals that mental handicap nursing has much in common with other contributing disciplines. This should be perceived as a strength rather than a weakness of its structure. No one has a franchise on knowledge, and it is knowledge which helps determine what contemporary mental handicap nursing is all about. The competent registered practitioner who is the product of the syllabus's aims and intentions will not perceive nursing care in a narrow way. She will know the available options which are necessary to make informed decisions. These decisions, based on competent practice, will assist in meeting the needs of the person who has a mental handicap in any setting. If the goal is reached, then others who genuinely have a commitment to appropriate and effective care of the person with a mental handicap should be willing to make their own contribution to this worthwhile process.

References

Chief Nursing Officer's Letter, *The Role of the Nurse in Caring for People with Mental Handicap*, DHSS CNO(85)5

English and Welsh National Boards for Nursing, Midwifery and Health Visiting, 'Syllabus of Training: Professional Register – Part 5 (Registered Nurse for the Mentally Handicapped)' 1982

English National Board for Nursing, Midwifery and Health Visiting, *Education and Training of Nurses Caring for People with Mental Handicap*, Circular 1985/55/ERDB 1985a

English National Board for Nursing, Midwifery and Health Visiting, *Caring for People with Mental Handicap—A Learning Package for Nurses* 1985b

Henderson, V., *The Nature of Nursing*, Collier—Macmillan, 1966

Rosenthal, N. and Jacobson, L. *Pygmalion in the Classroom*, Holt, Rinehart and Winston, 1968

Spencer, L. M., *Identifying, Measuring and Training Soft Skill Competencies*, McBer and Co., Boston, 1979

Chapter 2

Through my eyes—one nursing student's view

by Karen Morgan

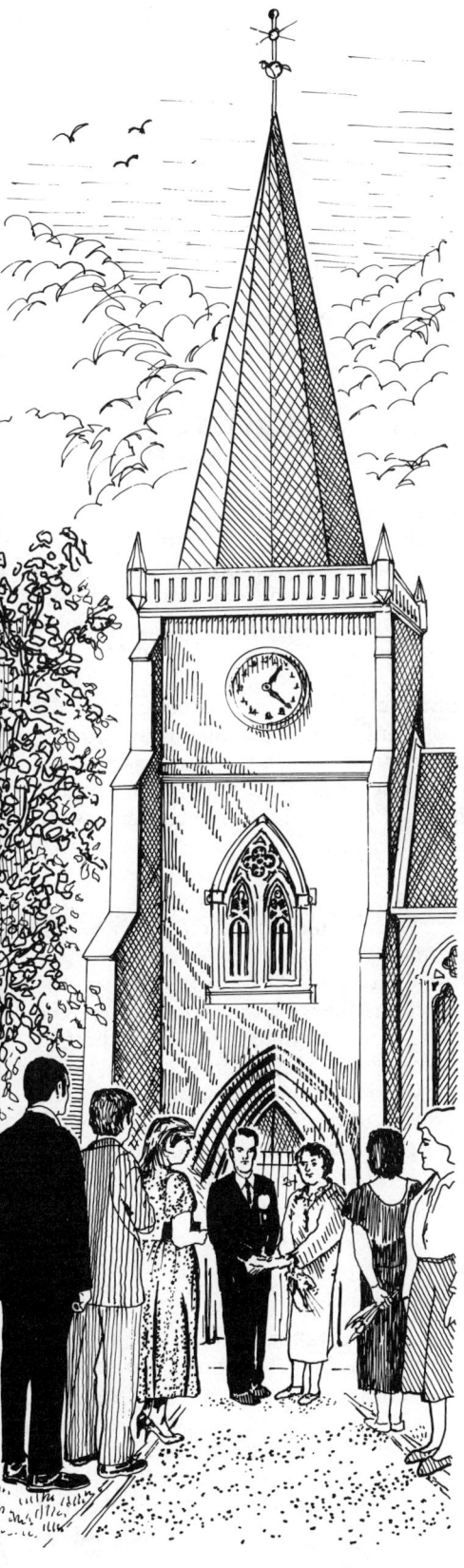

Becoming a student

Just two months away from the State final examination, I can reflect back (in between revision, of course) over the last three years to when it all began. Discontented with my job in drug research and development, I had applied to train in the field of mental handicap nursing. Without any insight or experience of mental handicap, I attended my interview.

I am ashamed to say that, as I entered the hospital grounds, I was terrified by all the 'disfigured, inhuman characters' I encountered. This now makes me realise how others, without knowledge and understanding, can develop ideas and fears about people with mental and physical handicaps, and how we as professionals can take on the role of public relations officers to untangle these ideas and alleviate the fears.

Much effort is made to bridge the gap between the hospital and its surrounding community. This is highlighted by the annual summer fair, a time when physical and mental handicaps become less apparent and the emphasis is on enjoyment.

Despite the good public relations work, there are still some staff who seem to enjoy exaggerating the story of a resident's violent outburst, in a loud voice, usually on public transport. Initially a breach of confidentiality, this also demonstrates a great disrespect for professionalism. Our professionalism depends upon our attitudes—to the person with mental handicap, to our work and to the other members of the caring team.

Attitudes serve to determine and guide our behaviour. It would, therefore, make sense to say that attitudes which are not geared to the currently adopted philosophy of 'normalisation' (Wolfensburger, 1972) could inhibit the achievement of individuality, rights, self-advocacy, choice and development for the person with mental handicap.

During my training, the attitudes of those I have worked with have been varied. Using the proverb 'Do unto others as you would have others do unto you' as my personal guide, I have attempted to learn more from those people whose attitudes I can accept, and to explain diplomatically, to those people whose attitudes I cannot accept, why our ideas conflict.

A good example of changing attitudes was the marriage between two mentally handicapped people after a forty-year relationship together. This was also an opportunity for the nurses involved to demonstrate their flexibility in changing roles, an idea instilled early in training. I was thrilled to be a bridesmaid, the ward sister naturally became mother of the bride and the clinical nurse specialist, continually stressing he was not old enough to be the bride's father, slipped into his new role with ease.

The day was perfect, an experience to be remembered fondly. There is a lesson to be learned from the dedication, loyalty and understanding that these two people have for one another, despite the restrictions imposed upon them by the institution in which they lived for so long.

Role play

The ability to adopt roles other than that of a nurse is important, especially today when we see so many changes in the field of mental handicap. Any distance between the resident and the nurse must be reduced, as the idea of not becoming personally involved is abandoned. For many residents, contact with family does not exist. These residents may then seek a family member substitute in a nurse.

I remember a ward sister, who was approaching retirement, asking me how many members there were in my family and how many friends I had. This puzzled me until she said; 'Is there any wonder we are so tired when we go home, after playing so many different roles for so many different people.'

Role play in school proved invaluable in my practical experiences, although at the time it was all giggles and red faces! Our personal tutor, who began teaching as we began our course, was very tolerant.

I am fortunate to be a member of a small but particularly close student group, which has meant additional support, guidance and encouragement, reinforced by the special relationship we have with our tutor. It was reassuring to know that once I had left the shelter of the nursing school, there would always be a tutor to whom I could return with any problems I might encounter.

Coping with frustrations

The biggest problem throughout my course has been the inability to put the theoretical ideals into practice. Staff shortages and the lack of resources are only partly to blame.

I have yet to meet a student who could claim to be supernumerary within her placement: instead there is a tendency to feel like 'an extra pair of hands', with learning needs often overlooked.

My first ward placement was typical—too many residents requiring a great deal of care and training and not enough members of staff to cope. However, I was quick to learn that it was not the *numbers* of staff that was important but the *qualities* that they possessed.

First there was the charge nurse, who terrified me. He knew how he wanted the ward run and what he wanted from his staff—a style of management, hovering between authoritarian and democratic, that obviously worked well. He would always throw me in at the deep end of any new situation, but was always there to ensure that I did not drown. I could rely on him to provide constructive criticism, and although he would never give verbal praise, you could sense his approval.

The morning medicine round at eight o'clock was a particularly nerve-racking experience. With a total lack of confidence, I would mumble and fumble my way through the practical side of it only to face a form of Spanish Inquisition, conducted by the charge nurse, who, it would seem, had previously swallowed the *British National Formulary*. (A year later I returned to the ward—of my own accord—so that the same nurse could conduct my drug assessment!)

At the time I felt I was learning through fear; now I realise it was because the charge nurse was such a good teacher. He wanted so much to share his knowledge and experience. I appreciate that.

The ward occupational therapist was a motherly lady protective of the residents and aware that I was still wary of them. She took the time to introduce me to them, telling me of their likes and dislikes, making me aware of the fact that they were all very individual people. I never felt silly asking her questions, whereas the nursing assistants, although it was never their intention, made me feel incompetent, unsure of what I was doing and self-conscious. They were always very efficient and thorough, knowing the ward routine and the hospital system. They also later turned out to be very good nursing students.

The evaluation process

The twelve-week placement went quickly; it had taken almost that time to settle and feel a part of the ward team. Now it was back to school, armed with an appraisal form and a wad of project work to prepare for another examination.

Now was the time to evaluate our placements. It would seem I had been one of the more fortunate students. Problems had already occurred with others, causing a reduction in the group's number. Some students had been resented by ward staff, as their presence had caused regular nurses to be 'booked out' to other wards. For some, support and guidance had been lacking, leaving students feeling overwhelmed, bewildered and isolated.

One thing had become apparent, however, even after such a short time: each of us had undergone some slight change in ourselves. Whether it was an increase in confidence, a more mature outlook, or gaining the ability to empathise, there was a two-way learning process occurring between us and the residents. While we were teaching them practical aspects of life to increase their independence, they were teaching us, among other things, to be patient, tolerant, sensitive and forgiving.

Moving towards the end of the first year, I found myself working with a ward sister who had the reputation of being 'a dragon'. I had been forewarned as to how I could expect to be treated and tipped how best to keep on her good side.

This was a fine example of how twisted and exaggerated stories can become within a hospital only to result in malicious and sometimes damaging gossip. The best way I found to ride the waves of gossip was to listen, never repeat, and only pass judgement or formulate opinions based on personal experience.

There was some element of truth in what was said about the sister, but I only had to work with her for six weeks before starting night duty. During my night duty experience I gave my first injection. I probably felt worse than the poor resident who was on the receiving end, but after carrying out the procedure my sense of achievement was so great that I felt my next step would be brain surgery!

The second year

Despite a good start to my training, I still suffered from the second-year 'blues'. It was a time when I felt neither here nor there. Pressures were beginning to mount. At work people were expecting more of me, as responsibilities and accountability increased. At home I was preparing to leave the security of my family and all the comforts taken for granted, to establish a new life with my fiancé, in a run-down old flat desperately needing attention. It was at this stage that I began to appreciate the difficulties and home-sickness that other students may have experienced, if they had had to leave home to begin the course.

Half of my group took up residence in the Nurses' Home, a very old and depressing building. They would complain of rooms 'not big enough to swing a cat in', with paper-thin walls, dirty, ill-equipped kitchens and clothes disappearing from the drying rooms. They had to contend with all-night parties. This was fine if you were a part of it, but beyond a joke if you were working the following early morning shift.

Living in the Nurses' Home meant that social life, more often than not, revolved around the hospital. I am not surprised they all found alternative accommodation eventually . . . .

Steadily gaining knowledge and confidence, I also felt myself losing interest and motivation. I was tired of making suggestions for training programmes and other forward-thinking techniques, when time and time again institutionalised staff would say: 'We tried that before, there is no point trying again, it will not work.' These people did not then realise that teaching a resident to feed himself, or to become continent, might take years of continually assessing, planning, implementing and evaluating several different approaches. They were willing to call it a day if no progress had been made within a matter of weeks after using inconsistent approaches.

With my ideas squashed and being pushed to one side as someone who was trying to create more work, I felt it was time to decide whether I would join their system, fight it or, easier still, leave it altogether and go for a steady nine-to-five job, that paid better wages and gave me evenings and weekends free, with holidays when *I* wanted to take them. I chose to fight on for the final year.

The third year

Towards the final examination it was necessary to have experience for nine weeks in the local general hospital. To tell the truth, I did not expect to be able to walk the length of the designated medical ward without passing out: to say I was squeamish would be an understatement! As a group, our expectations of this placement were much the same. The 'proper' general nurses would be aloof and look down on us, questioning our nurse status and wondering why we had to complete three years of training only to end up feeding residents and washing them! We imagined that we would be treated as outsiders and left to fulfil the simple tasks of running to and fro with bedpans and commodes. Oh, how wrong we were! It was exactly the opposite. Obviously I had watched too many American movies, where blood, pain and rushing around saving lives was the order of the day. As for the nurses, they welcomed us and made us feel very much at home. They showed respect for our work in the field of mental handicap and were eager to learn from us, to the extent of asking us to conduct teaching sessions on subjects such as epilepsy. In turn, they gave us every opportunity to obtain general nursing skills.

Coping with death

However, there was one skill I could not master: the ability to cope with death. This was a subject that the studies had not yet covered, leaving us ill-prepared. The first death I encountered occurred while I was on my own with the patient. This death was expected, as disseminated carcinoma had been diagnosed, but I still felt I needed to put my feelings on to paper—probably a gesture considered silly by others.

I watch from the end of the bed, frightened to approach.
Dying, is this what it is all about?
Would I like to wave goodbye to someone who is not there,
Or cruise the world alone?
Hardly a comparison to this lonely end.
I could turn my back and return when it was over.
Instead I reach for the hand, cold and pale,
And return the gaze that I hope can see the caring
    human being I am,
And not the removed, unemotional professional I am
    thought to be.
I talk softly but do you want to hear?
Or shall I sit in silence while you recall treasured
    memories.
What terrible crime did you commit to deserve this
    cruel sentence?
'Is there anything you want?'
I ask, like an executioner allowing you a final request.
You left without answering.
I'm sorry, these tears are not for you
But for those you leave behind.
Life is a precious gift, received without thanks.

(January, 1985)

Experience in the community

This is where, I had been led to believe, it was all happening! *Care in the community is the care of the future.* With all the large institutions gradually closing down, according to the NHS Regional Strategic Plans, the residents are being put back to the places they were originally plucked from, sometimes as long as seventy years ago. Whether this is right or wrong (and there are arguments for and against community care), we are preparing our residents as best we can with the resources available.

While preparing our residents for the community, we should also consider preparing the community for our residents. After all, everyone will suffer if the general public refuse to accept and acknowledge our residents' right to a place in the mainstream of society.

It must be remembered that it is not only the hospitals for the mentally handicapped that are closing, but also those for the mentally ill.

Our community mental handicap team has been established for several years and serves, among other functions, to assist in settling residents and monitoring their welfare when they are in the community. The team is still relatively small in numbers, consisting of nurses and social workers, working together within the team's headquarters. It therefore surprised me to discover that as well as caring for those people leaving the hospital, they were also responsible for the care received by approximately one thousand people who were already in the community, living on their own or with their families.

It became apparent that community life was not entirely a bed of roses and not necessarily the answer to the problems of the institutions. Resources here were also stretched to their limits, with many families pressurised and suffering, owing to receiving little or no help. To see a family torn apart because aged parents could no longer cope with a severely handicapped son, but felt too guilty to place him in another home, or too proud to admit they desperately needed time to themselves, was very disturbing.

However, in fairness to community life, there are also the happy stories, like the seventy-five-year-old lady, who as she walked out of the hospital gates to begin a life in the community said: 'I never thought I would walk out of this prison. I always thought I would leave in a box.' Quite a statement for someone who was supposed to be mentally handicapped!

Many of the homes to which the residents will go are controlled by Social Services and are staffed by people not all of whom are necessarily qualified to work with people who are mentally handicapped. This is not necessarily wrong, for there is a great deal of good work going on, but as mental handicap nurses we should be prepared to defend our nurse status and convince others that the specialised skills acquired during our professional education have a very important place in the community. To secure our future, we must believe that we are the right people to lead the movement that will ensure a better standard of living for the mentally handicapped person.

The sceptics who say that we are institutionalised and therefore only capable of functioning in such a place must be shown that we are not frightened of change and progression.

In 1979 the Jay Report recommended that mental handicap nursing should be phased out to make way for a new model of care. Today Project 2000 recognises the need to retain specialised areas of nursing after a period of common foundation work has been completed.

Nursing courses are already undergoing revision and this has come in the form of the new 1982 syllabus. It means that the majority of time for future students will be spent in the community, so I hope it will encourage those professions out there, who do not yet appear to understand the role of nurses and their preparation, to become familiar with nursing education and the opportunities it offers.

I have been asked by social workers, teachers of special education and physiotherapists what it is I do that other professions working for the mentally handicapped are not already doing. With tongue in cheek I have replied, 'everything they do put together, only with a greater understanding of the person as a whole'.

Professional responsibility

During my third year I came face to face with my biggest dilemma yet. In the past there had been instances where I had witnessed procedures I was not happy with, such as the degradation of residents by mass bathing, not unlike 'sheep dipping'. Now I had witnessed the deliberate sick mistreatment of a resident by a member of staff.

I had always suppressed my guilt and the internal conflict I felt when I followed instructions of doubtful propriety. Continual rationalisation meant that I never challenged what I was being told to do; after all I was new to the system; I needed a good report.(!) However, mistreatment of the resident was something conscience could not overlook. I knew that reporting the incident would result in serious consequences. When it came to the crunch, although I reported what I had seen, I was unable to name the member of staff concerned. As a result, in some ways I felt I had let the resident involved down, as he was unable to speak and defend his own interests.

I have always maintained that if I had not spoken out, it would have been a farce to continue calling myself a nurse. After all, a nurse is someone who is educated to care.

The matter was dealt with and I heard no more. I was not victimised as I expected to be, although all the while I had considered myself a trouble maker, to be labelled accordingly for the future.

The above is an example of the nurse as an advocate. However, it is not possible for so few nurses to be advocates for so many residents. An attempt to overcome this problem has been made by 'Advocacy Alliance', where volunteers are trained to become advocates in order that they may assist an individual to achieve a higher quality of life.

The only advocate I have encountered (not necessarily typical of all advocates) had all the best intentions but saw the staff as a threat to her cause. The nursing staff were happy to co-operate and pass on their knowledge of the resident the advocate was representing, but this was interpreted as interference. It was only after the advocate had taken the resident on a week's holiday that the practical difficulties of caring for a person both physically and mentally handicapped were fully appreciated. The relationship between the advocate and the nurses then improved.

Nearing the end of my three years, I was now taking charge of wards. In one respect I was enjoying this: it was giving me more job satisfaction and testing my confidence. In another respect, I felt used, just a form of cheap labour temporarily to replace a staff nurse or ward sister.

When it came to the drug round, I required, by law, a qualified nurse to supervise me. In the beginning I was stupid enough to suppose that higher management would arrange this. In the end I would have to telephone other wards, literally begging for a nurse to supervise my round, as management had either forgotten I was on my own or had instructed me to do the telephoning around. The fact that support did not seem to be present for the routine requirements made me wonder whether it would be there in an emergency. When I spoke out, no one appeared to notice my concern over the lack of support student nurses were receiving while running a ward. When I rebelled by going absent without notification, I may have received an informal warning, but I also made my point. Students can now expect more support!

The future

Enough now of the past. What of the present? Here I am with the end in sight, feeling slightly uncertain of what the future may hold for me.

My final placement, by choice, will last nearly five months, giving me the opportunity to settle and absorb the lessons in management I am receiving from my present ward sister.

I am pleased to be working alongside other students, some of them very junior, for I feel partly responsible for them. My increased empathy with them, I hope, will make me more approachable if they should have any problems, and if they do begin to lack encouragement, support or guidance, I hope my own experiences will enable me to recognise their needs. I sometimes think a student only feels truly understood by another student . . . .

The state final examination has now been and gone and the outcome was that of success. I cannot help feeling proud of my achievement but at the same time thankful and grateful to all those people who helped me along the way, especially my husband Dave.

My student days are still far from over, for I am now studying general nursing at Normanby College, King's Health District. I do not consider that I have abandoned my cause in mental handicap nursing: instead I feel I am spreading a greater understanding of our speciality into another area of our profession. I also feel that certain specialised skills such as communication, the ability to empathise and understand an individual as a whole person, are sometimes lacking in general nursing. By being able to offer these skills, I am a valuable asset to nursing and hopefully will help to gain further recognition and respect for all those trained in the field of mental handicap nursing, whether they have trained under the pre-1982 syllabus, as I have done, or are at present training under the recently implemented 1982 syllabus.

Reference

Wolfensburger, W., *Normalisation*, National Institute of Mental Retardation, Toronto, 1972

Chapter 3

Human rights and mental handicap

by Alison Morton-Cooper

Introduction

The aim of this chapter is not to provide you with a run-down of the legal, moral or political rights of the person with a mental handicap; rather, the written and oral exercises are intended as a means for you to explore and examine your own attitudes and beliefs regarding mental handicap, as you have come into contact with it.

By studying some of the practical dilemmas and difficulties experienced by people and families affected by limitations brought about by mental handicap, you should become more adept at recognising situations where your own clients' rights may at present be denied, or not fully realised.

What we expect of a civilised society

'All human beings are born free and equal in dignity and rights . . . '
(*Universal Declaration of Human Rights*, Article 1, 1948)

If the principles of this *Declaration*, adopted by the member countries of the United Nations in 1948, were today a reality rather than an ideal, there would probably be no need to discuss such matters in a chapter such as this. However, decisions which directly concern human rights are sometimes made even before a human being comes into the world. By virtue of certain kinds of handicap, detected *in utero*, some babies are never born at all in Western countries, as the parents, with the consent and counsel of medical advisers, may exercise their right to have the pregnancy terminated.

Perhaps a mother has come into contact with rubella and has become seriously infected, or she has conceived the child while taking drugs or other substances which are known to be harmful to the developing fetus. An amniocentesis test in an older mother may have detected a chromosomal abnormality in the child, known as Down's Syndrome.

In the United Kingdom the lobby to protect the life of the unborn child is strong, but so, too, is the lobby which protects the parents' right to choose whether or not they should give birth to a child which will in all probability be born 'handicapped'.

Questions will be asked about whether a fetus is viable. Will it survive the trauma of birth? If it does, what are its chances of survival thereafter? How will the parents cope with their child? Who will take responsibility for him and his future?

It could be said that, once the child has been conceived, it is already subject to human rights: that it has a *right to be born*. But does this therefore mean that obstetricians, parents or others who condone abortion for any reason are already infringing the rights of the child, regardless of whether it is born handicapped or not? What about the health and personal circumstances of the mother? What about the kind of future this child can reasonably expect?

Exercise 1

Arrange a debate to be held in class and see who poses the strongest and most convincing argument. Your debate could be entitled: 'No child should be denied the right to be born, whatever the circumstances of its parents, or its viability'. An alternative title might be: 'Every woman has the right to choose whether or not she should give birth to a child which is expected to be born mentally or physically imperfect'.

It won't have taken you long to discover that there is no clear answer to this debate. Next, consider the child which is born unexpectedly handicapped. What choices may be made on his or her behalf and by whom? Every child is born dependent on its parents and others for food, comfort and protection. Should we assume that the handicapped child is equally as dependent as or more dependent than the non-handicapped child, and, if so, how long will this greater degree of dependence last, compared with that of the non-handicapped child?

A civilised society may be distinguished from an uncivilised one by its attitude to its dependent members. If it was advocated that all fetuses suspected of having a severe handicap should be aborted, or that every child born with a severe handicap should be suffocated at birth, what do you suppose the attitude of the general public might be? Sympathy with the view, or moral outrage?

Discuss this with your fellow students and see whether you can reach a consensus of opinion.

Examining attitudes and beliefs

A study of attitudes towards people with Down's Syndrome undertaken by Sinson in 1985 showed a mixed response from a largely ignorant and apprehensive public. Sinson investigated attitudes to Down's Syndrome in urban and rural Yorkshire and compared the attitudes of people in the towns with those in more rural areas. If the results of her study are representative of the British attitude as a whole, then the earlier supposition that we are living in a civilised country may be seriously called into question.

When asked what should happen to the father of Louise Brown (a Down's baby), who was at that time awaiting trial accused of her murder, parents in the survey were often ambivalent. Twenty-six per cent of mothers felt that even if Mr Brown were found guilty of his handicapped daughter's murder, he should not be punished as severely as if he had murdered a non-handicapped child.

Typical comments included:

'I think he killed the child to put it out of its misery.'
'. . . not as severely as if he'd murdered a normal child.'
'Well, say if it was me, I couldn't cope. I believe that if you think the child's going to be happier not here—you've got the right to kill it.'

Exercise 2

How prevalent is this view in your experience? From a sample of your own acquaintances and friends conduct a small survey of attitudes to the same question. Try to read Sinson's study in full, so that you have a clear idea of the controls used in this kind of study.

You will probably have already received guidance on the many causes of mental handicap and the nature of the disabilities it can bring about. Try asking your sample (as above) what they think actually *causes* mental handicap. Compare their views with the medical definitions you have been given previously as part of your nursing education.

Would you consider the people involved in your study to be knowledgeable or ignorant on the whole? What factors do you suppose influence their acquired knowledge and beliefs?

Key concepts in carer advocacy

The following exercise is designed to help you identify your own attitudes to certain concepts as they are applied to your professional work situation. Carry out the first part of it on your own, but report back to other students in your group who have asked themselves the same questions. It may be useful to appoint a class member to act as an observer (making notes and observations on the way you use body language—posture, inflection of voice, expression of hands, touch, and so on) when you report your answers back verbally to the assembled class.

Exercise 3

Working on your own, see whether you can define the words or concepts in Table 3.1, without a dictionary if possible. It is important to set yourself a time limit: about two minutes per definition would be about right.

Table 3.1 Key concepts in carer advocacy

Normal	Progress
Abnormal	Advocacy
Decision-making	Responsibility
Institution	Patronise
Institutionalised	Do-gooding
Representation	Morality
Patronage	Exploitation
Person	Patient
Dignity	Client
Platitudes	Community

Now compare your definitions with those arrived at by your fellow students and see whether you can identify where the main differences lie. Did your observer notice anything in particular about the way you put your arguments across?

How confident were you? Which words or concepts proved most difficult to define? Have you altered your own definition or attitude to a concept as a result of anything said in class? If you have, make sure you note it down for reference purposes later.

It will probably become apparent that each of us has a slightly different concept of our roles as carers. If we all have individual ideas about the way we should deliver care to our clients, should we suppose that our clients, too, have strong views on the way care is delivered and received?

Have you ever been in a situation, for example, where you have been in danger of doing things 'to' and 'for' a client when he might have preferred to 'do' and 'be' for himself, albeit less expertly?

At a seminar on *Better Living for Mentally Handicapped People* (Banga, 1985) one nurse made a special plea to those involved in caring for people with such a handicap. Having referred to a book which discussed the materialism of *having*, as opposed to the spiritual qualities of *being*, she said she saw 'improving the quality of being' as her aim as carer. 'It means improving the quality of life and giving people the right to be human with choices in unregimented environments. Being warm, fed and clothed is not enough', she said. She also suggested that conflicts invariably arose when considering the morality and 'rightness' of community care for this 'hitherto neglected section of society', often as a result of unresolved questions. She stressed the need to address these questions.

Perhaps what she was trying to say is that too often the carers themselves impose their own views and values on their clients, rather than asking them what they want or need. Unresolved questions about our roles and our attitudes, as well as those of our clients, have to be resolved before we can hope to help the person with a mental handicap exercise his rights as an individual in a society which has yet to accept him as an equal, with the same freedoms, rights and privileges as any other citizen who respects and lives according to the laws of his country.

An exploration of human rights

Working as a group, read through the following list.

Every human being has the right to:

- Be born, and have access to all life-saving expertise and technology.
- Be loved and accepted unconditionally.
- Be given adequate warmth, food and shelter according to his need.

- Express himself verbally, physically, culturally, emotionally and sexually.
- Be educated.
- Work.
- Worship.
- Make choices and, where necessary, mistakes.
- Choose where he lives and with whom.
- Experience human emotion directly (e.g. pain, pleasure, hurt, anxiety, rejection, anger, grief, anguish, humour, love, affection, loss, jealousy, loyalty . . .).
- Marry and have children.
- Take responsibility for himself and others.
- Enjoy the companionship of friends and the family group.
- Belong to a peer group.
- Explore and discover the world outside his own home.
- Representation on all legal, political and constitutional matters (especially to vote at a general election).
- Live according to the laws of his country or accept the consequences of failure to do so.
- Freedom of speech and movement within the law.

Are there any rights which you consider inappropriate for a person with a mental handicap? If your answer is 'yes', discuss why. If you think that all of these rights are unassailable and therefore 'go without saying', go over each one again and think about how practical it would be for you to exercise these rights as an able-bodied and intelligent person.

Consider how easy it would be for a mentally handicapped person. Who has the most difficulty, you or your client? What are the social and political factors which affect his ability to exercise these rights in the light of his nationality, his personal circumstances and the attitudes of those in positions of power and influence, such as local government officers or officials?

Can you identify the nature of the prejudices or fears which might prevent your client from exercising his rights fully? More importantly, how can we create a climate for change so that barriers to progress may be broken down and a more sympathetic and understanding attitude engendered in and by the communities in which we live?

Dealing with prejudices and fears

It could be argued that the large mental handicap hospitals which have evolved over the last 150 years came about as a result of society's inability to cope with the socially unacceptable behaviour (as seen in some people with a mental handicap) or indeed the consequences of it. The notion that all mentally handicapped individuals behave in a socially unacceptable or distasteful manner is still held by sections of the community, even though they may have had very little direct experience of or contact with a handicapped person.

The human mind has an age-old method of dealing with something it finds unacceptable: 'I will put it away and think no more about it.' This is manifest in the poor and degrading conditions in some of Britain's inner cities, in its overcrowded and often insanitary prisons, and, tragically, in a few of the mental handicap hospitals which await their share of limited cash resources to be updated and made fit for human habitation.

Medical science and public morals have progressed since the inception of the Welfare State, but for many it is assumed that the National Health Service will take full responsibility, abdicating the citizen's obligation to help the individual with a disability to as normal and full a life as possible in a home of his own. Mental disability is seen as 'the government's problem'—an attitude which fosters negative feelings and a resistance to the idea that a person with a mental handicap (or illness) can live and work in the community the same as you or I.

However, it is not only mentally handicapped people who meet with such indifference or outright prejudice. What about the schoolboy with haemophilia who returned to school having been diagnosed as a carrier of the AIDS virus? Why did the parents of his classmates refuse to send their children back to school, despite assurances from the DHSS that it was perfectly safe to do so? Was it a result of ignorance and fear over what might happen if their own children came into contact with the boy, or of lack of confidence in the education and health authorities that 'they knew what they were doing'?

It is not difficult, by the careful and studied use of alarmist language and a sense of moral outrage, for the press and media to capitalise on the fears and uncertainties of their readers and viewers/listeners. Although it may not always be a conscious decision, editors, when looking for a 'good story', will seek out an 'angle' or approach to a story which has the best chance of capturing the reader's attention, perhaps one that will cause a considerable sensation among the public.

There are generally two sides to a story about 'dependent' members of our society (usually children, elderly people and mentally handicapped people). The contentious 'Old Woman Evicted from Council Flat after 50 Happy Years' or 'Handicapped Child Left to Fend for Herself while Dad Drinks in Pub' are guaranteed to win sympathy and arouse a sense of moral indignation in the reader.

The other well-meaning but somewhat patronising approach may be 'Disabled Kids Succeed where Others Fail'. You or I might say: why shouldn't they? They entered the race to win, didn't they? A recent story in a national quality newspaper reported that 'three paraplegics' raised money for charity. Had the money been raised by individuals who were not paraplegic, do you suppose that the story would have read: 'Three men raised money for charity'? Almost certainly not! At the very least, the reader would have been given details of the men's names, their ages, and where they lived and worked.

Individuals are very skilled at labelling or categorising people: pigeonholing them into acceptable compartments so that certain social rules and customs may be strictly adhered to. If, for instance, you were at a party and the stranger next to you asked you what you did for a living, what would you say? If you said you were a psychiatrist, what might he reply? If you said you were a breeder of budgerigars (no disrespect to such people intended), do you suppose he would pursue the same line of conversation?

The following are examples of labelling. They can be heard daily in hospitals and doctors' surgeries throughout the UK.

OAPs
The chronic sick
Geriatrics
The working class
The antenatals
The breast on the surgical unit
The mentally handicapped

Discuss whether or not you think it is reasonable to define groups of people in this way. Is it any different from describing people as 'city-dwellers', for instance, or as 'commuters' or 'rail passengers'? If you believe that labelling is detrimental to our view of people as individuals, what would you suggest as an alternative means of identifying people? How do we avoid labelling and categorising people and yet still manage to describe groups of people in our communities in an acceptable and fair way?

For most of us, labelling is just another way of conforming. If you would like to see just how powerful the human instinct to conform is, try walking along a busy street. Stop suddenly and look up at some imaginary object in the sky. Stay where you are and keep staring. Within five minutes you will have gathered an inquisitive crowd behind you who are all prepared to Ooh! and Aah! with you at that same imaginary object!

Educating ourselves to care constructively

If we are to hope to change our own and the public's response to the dilemmas experienced by our mentally handicapped clients, we must first deal with our own prejudices and fears. The recognition of rights such as those outlined above depends on several very important preconditions:

- A desire on the part of members of a community to see that change is brought about.
- That a means of educating people about their rights exists and is used to capacity.
- That there exists a means of preventing the vulnerable individual from being exploited for material or personal gain (such as theft of benefits,

abuse of the franchise for political ends, unlawful sexual intercourse or assault, dishonest landlords, etc.).

- That adequate resources are available to develop social and welfare services in response to need, and that these are run efficiently.
- That a means of fair representation of the views of the person with a mental handicap exists electorally and personally.
- That society believes that a person with a mental handicap may be capable of making his own decisions and is able to act on them accordingly.

The concept of a nurse or doctor as 'custodian' is now largely outmoded, and due recognition of the fact that most clients *can* exercise their right to choose is becoming more acceptable and usual. The most powerful barrier to the exercise of that right has often been the custodian's or guardian's habit of making choices on behalf of the person for whom he or she is caring. In the past the attitude has been: 'I will choose for you because I do not believe that you are capable of making that choice for yourself.' Not only has this actively prevented any exercise of basic rights for the mentally handicapped person, but also it has absolved the carer from having to educate his client as to what his choices actually are. Rather than examine the possibilities of a course of action in detail (such as 'where I will live and with whom'), it has been arbitrarily decided that 'here is a ward or room and you shall live in it, for society does not expect otherwise'.

It is not difficult to see why both professional carers and their clients have become institutionalised in the past. Neither is it difficult to see that a change of basic attitude could substantially improve the chances of human rights being recognised and exercised fully.

It has always been a criticism of the caring professions that we have too often based our actions on what we think would 'be good for the client or patient' to the best of *our* knowledge and beliefs rather than *theirs*. Perhaps now is the time to reconsider that view, and to ask ourselves why we are the people making some of the decisions, when instead we could be finding out what our clients want. Instead of clinging to the custodial kind of advocacy which was expected of us in the past, we could now be forging ahead to assist clients in obtaining the information and wherewithal to make decisions for themselves, albeit we might not agree with their decision or approve of the outcome.

We jealously guard our own right to make successes or failures of what we do with our lives: it must be progress to assist our clients in doing the same. There are many other rights which cannot be gone into here but which could bear much closer examination. These include:

- The right to privacy.
- The right to make mistakes.
- The right to belong.
- The right to live, work and die in dignity and peace.

It would be wrong to give the impression that to be without handicap presupposes that instantly all our human rights are recognised and respected. What about the child born to parents who are violent or negligent? What about the unemployed person? What about the young school-leaver who has no skills and grave concerns for his ability to earn his own living? What about the innocent victims of civil riot or political oppression?

Educating ourselves to care constructively must mean helping one another to independence as far as is humanly possible. Human dignity has no limitations, save those which we seek to impose on one another by our attitudes and expectations, and by the way we express our concerns for one another *to* one another. Independence and self-respect are the rocks on which human dignity is founded. Without our self-respect we feel less valued, less esteemed and, most crucial of all, less needed.

If we as human beings (unlabelled and uncategorised!) can impress upon one another that we are all equally needed and loved, and that no conditions are attached to that love, then we have respected the most fundamental of all human rights in this world: the right simply *to be*.

References

D. Banga, *Better Living for People with Mental Handicap*, report of a seminar by the North West Herts Community Health Council with the Council for Voluntary Service St Albans and District, June 1985

J. C. Sinson, *Attitudes to Down's Syndrome—An Investigation of Attitudes to Mental Handicap in Urban and Rural Yorkshire,* Mental Health Foundation, London, 1985

Further reading

Campbell, A. V., *Moderated Love—A Theology of Professional Care*, SPCK, 1984

Campbell, T., Goldberg, D., McLean, S. and Mullen, T., *Human Rights—From Rhetoric to Reality*, Blackwell, 1986

Getting Together—Sexual and Social Expression for Mentally Handicapped People, Mind Publications, Harley Street, London, 1982

Hebden, J., *She'll Never Do Anything, Dear*, Human Horizons Special, Souvenir Press, 1985

Lockwood, M. (ed.), *Moral Dilemmas in Modern Medicine*, Oxford University Press, 1985

McConkey, R. and McCormack, R., *Breaking Barriers—Educating People about Disability*, Human Horizon Series, Souvenir Press, 1983

McGilloway, O. and Myco, F. (eds), *Nursing and Spiritual Care*, Lippincott Nursing Series, Harper and Row, 1985 [see especially Chapter 13, 'Spiritual Care in Mental Handicap']

Sutherland, A. T., *Disabled We Stand*, Human Horizons Series, Souvenir Press, 1981

Walsh, J., *Let's Make Friends*, Human Horizon Series, Souvenir Press, 1986

Chapter 4 A close look at relationships
by Amanda Gunner

Have you ever wondered why something as fundamental as the understanding of human relationships is often left to chance, while we are taught how to read and write in a formalised environment? The way we perceive relationships is usually based upon what we have learnt throughout our lives, together with specific experiences we may have had. The pages which follow will look at:

- The nature of relationships, with whom we have them, how we respond to them and how strategies may be developed for coping with them.
- The myths which can surround people who are mentally handicapped and their ability to enjoy and develop relationships.
- Why people with a mental handicap are at risk of 'missing out' with regard to personal relationships.

Before we consider relationships and people who are mentally handicapped, the following exercises will set the scene by clarifying for the reader what the term 'relationships' means.

Exercise

What is a relationship and what do you expect from and give to it?
Think about the above question for a few minutes; then write down your answer on a separate sheet of paper. There is no right answer, but the question is something on which we all have ideas.

Brainstorming exercise

Who are those with whom we have relationships?
1. On a separate sheet of paper write down any thoughts that come to mind in relation to the above question.
2. Look at your list. Are you able to group your answers so that a pattern emerges, showing the types of relationships we have?
   i.e. intimate <————————> superficial?

Living in today's world, relationships (particularly personal relationships) are viewed as symbols of success. The media constantly bombard us with answers on how to strive for the ideal. Advertising, with its suggestive overtones, pressures us into believing that success is synonymous with being cared for and loved. Those who cannot to a greater or lesser extent compete in the relationships game, because of partial or severe disability, may find themselves rejected as non-starters. Society is unable to cope with the idea that disabled people have the same needs and desires as themselves.

> 'And by society I do not mean just the ordinary able-bodied person who has little or no contact with his handicapped neighbour: what is more shaking and more serious is to find this attitude widespread amongst those who are intimately involved through their treatment and care of the disabled in their homes or in residential situations.' (Greengross, 1976)

Relationships of all kinds are based upon communication. This need to communicate with other human beings in one way or another can be restricted for people who are mentally handicapped, because of the protected environment in which they live and sometimes the nature of their own particular circumstances.

Society sometimes regards such people as having 'no sense—no feelings', believing that 'they' do not need to know about such sophisticated things as relationships. Because mentally handicapped people are different, they may be viewed as disgusting, indecent or even comic when wishing to express their own personal feelings.

This reaction may be partly due to the myth, subconsciously perpetrated, that individuals who are handicapped will give birth to similarly handicapped children and therefore flood the population with individuals who will undermine the whole basis of society — an almost wholly inaccurate assumption! The study reported by Reed and Reed (1965), into parents with mental handicaps, is one of the most comprehensive on this subject.

Perhaps the reactions of those who are not disabled are really a reflection of their feelings about their own relationships. If they are personally unable to sustain a high level of satisfaction in a relationship, then there is less chance of success for a person with a mental handicap, whom they may consider to be inferior anyway. It is not uncommon for parents of children without handicaps to try to ignore that their children are growing up into adulthood. As a result children may respond in 'adolescent rebellion', with sexuality and sex itself becoming a potential weapon and certainly a source of angst and worry to the family generally.

Not all relationships need to be of a social nature. Friendship begins for most people within the family. The majority of people with a mental handicap have been or still are cared for at home by their families. And while the family unit may provide the love and care needed by the person as an individual, this in itself can create problems of conflict. For instance, the mother who becomes totally devoted to the care of her handicapped child may unintentionally neglect or ignore other members of the family (sibling rivalry).

The mentally handicapped child may receive an otherwise disproportionate amount of attention from his parents, leaving little or no time for other children in the family, who also have needs, even though they may differ considerably from those of the first child. The guilt of the parents towards their handicapped child can effectively stifle him, and starve his brothers and sisters of fulfilment of their needs, which may go partly or wholly unrecognised. Having been left to their own devices, other children may well become resentful — and this feeling can build up, with potentially harmful consequences to sibling relationships and to the stability of the family as a whole.

Dilemmas facing the family

Let us assume that coupled with friendship is loyalty. Within society, loyalty towards the family is viewed with the utmost importance. Any child who has somehow been neglected, either emotionally or physically, because his family only considered their handicapped child is likely to develop a conflict of loyalty towards his family. In desperation he may look outside the family for comfort and fulfilment of his own unmet needs. This situation can be complicated further if his handicapped brother or sister realises the conflict.

Ignoring the pressure put upon the child, who, in becoming aware of his need for mutually satisfying relationships, feels angry or guilty because help and understanding is lacking, is a denial of his rights as a human being. On the other hand, caring for an individual who is mentally handicapped requires a constant devotion which most parents might feel unable to give or even contemplate. Tolerance of the attitude of parents and the dilemmas which face them — i.e. their 'shutting their eyes and hoping problems will go away' — should be understood, not criticised or condemned out of hand. The often taken for granted pleasures of extending a circle of friends and exploring and developing feelings towards people outside of the family can often be denied to the mentally handicapped person because he may be over-protected by those who care for him, or because of segregation as a result of the sheltered environment in which he lives.

Today's philosophy of Normalisation (Wolfensburger, 1972) should no longer disadvantage persons with a mental handicap. The very ethos of Normalisation is about the way you treat people, *not* how to be 'normal'. The principles of normalisation are that:

- People with a mental handicap have the same human value as anyone else.
- Such people have a right and a need to live like others in their community.
- Services must recognise the individuality of mentally handicapped people.

The emphasis in today's world is upon the rights of the individual as a consumer of goods or services, be it buying a car, receiving treatment from a general practitioner or being able to live as an individual within a community (See Chapter 3). So why do people with a mental handicap continue to miss out on aspects of life which the rest of society views as a right? As already discussed, the fears of parents are that their children may be exploited through friendships (deemed to be 'the wrong sort of company') or sexually abused, while society sees intellectually impaired people as childlike and vulnerable, and in need of 'protection'.

Additional stress may be placed on the mentally handicapped individual when a relationship is formed and valued, and then brought to an abrupt end: for example, the death of a relative; a fellow resident moves from hospital; or a member of staff whom he trusts and likes moves jobs or is transferred to another unit or hospital.

Bereavement

Every one of us experiences loss at some time in our lives. The most traumatic and final can be the loss of a close relative or much-loved friend. For anyone, bereavement may cause a number of reactions: disbelief about what has happened, anger, depression, fear, exhaustion, loss of appetite, inability to concentrate, aggression or sleep disturbance.

Some or all of these reactions are a natural part of the human grieving process, and they may last for many weeks or months, disappearing only to return without warning as the memory is jogged by a particular sound, sight or smell. Such reactions may be seen by others or may only emerge in privacy.

To suppose that a person with a mental handicap will not experience any of these emotions would be naive, unkind and possibly harmful to the bereaved person. Instead it should be recognised that such a person may even have additional special difficulties due to:

1. Poor intellect and multiple disabilities which may deny him the many social, verbal, auditory and visual opportunities of realising and coming to terms with the death as more able people would.
2. The failure of professionals and others to recognise grief and the individual's response to it.

No two individuals respond to loss in exactly the same way. The grieving process should be recognised and respected as a natural defence mechanism which has evolved in order to allow people to cope with and survive what could otherwise be an intolerable experience. Nurses should be sympathetic and watchful for any additional problems which may complicate the process by virtue of the restrictions and special difficulties brought about by mental handicap for the person in their care.

(a) Loss of the parental home

The loss of a parent or parents to a dependent person may necessitate many potentially disturbing changes in his life-style and habits. A move into residential care may become necessary and this may be some distance from the parental home. The familiar neighbourhood will have to be left behind, and perhaps the day centre the person knew so well, with familiar friends and staff. The security of what has perhaps been a daily routine for many years may be sacrificed, and contact with relatives and friendly neighbours may be lost or threatened.

If the bereaved person is known to the statutory social services, then such a wrench may be avoided, although this will greatly depend on professionals' sensitivity to the situation and knowledge of the family. Failure to recognise grief can inadvertently lead to the bereaved person exhibiting so-called 'difficult' behaviour and so being labelled a 'problem' client.

Consider the situation of a family where the affected person is supported by ageing parents. If the family is not known to the statutory social services until the death of one or other of his parents, then he could be put in the position of requiring emergency residential care and subsequent long-term support. If the worst happened and the bereaved person had to leave home and suddenly become surrounded by strangers in a new and strange place, with only a cursory explanation as to what has happened to his deceased relative, then his chances of recovering from the experience are substantially reduced, and he is placed at increased risk emotionally and psychologically.

Inappropriate judgements of care requirements can lead to the person exhibiting withdrawn and apathetic behaviour of a type which leads to 'learned helplessness', as described by Seligman (1975). The individual needs of the person should be regarded as paramount by carers, regardless of the care setting or the routine of daily work.

(b) The nurse's role

Whether within the residential setting or in the community at large, those caring for people with a mental handicap will become aware of the potential problems raised by grieving. Copperman (1983) states that people need help in coping with grief, and this is a part of preventive health care.

The loss of a family member through death is not the only time when a bereavement can occur. For a person living in residential care, friendships may be lost or curtailed because of people moving away. To a mentally handicapped person this loss can be as traumatic as loss through death.

The combination of a new philosophy and more enlightened social policies has, for the good of those people with a mental handicap, decided that care in the community is the optimum model of care. Even for those who have lived in large institutions all their lives, radical change is proposed. A move, perhaps to a pre-hostel environment, may be considered where the person may learn and improve upon domestic skills. A home in the community, either alone (with support) or with other fellows 'sharing' independence, may be the eventual goal.

For others, however, delays and scarcity of money to fund moves into the community may mean a ward closure in line with the Health Authority's strategic plan, and this may mean transfer to a different ward or even a different institution. Any of the situations mentioned above may mean loss of friendships and contacts. Familiar environments and activities may also be lost.

Exposure to new and strange surroundings can arouse feelings of insecurity. A loss of confidence as to how to cope could therefore be expected as a 'natural outcome' to this. To help clients overcome this anxious time, staff should be supportive, allowing time for emotions to be shown and for a settling-down period to be gone through. It would be impossible to estimate how long such a phase should take, but if handled sensitively and at the pace of the individual client, reasonable progress should be made possible.

(c) Staff changes

Changes in staff due to rotation, shift patterns and status may also lead to a period of loss for both nurses and clients. While it is generally accepted that nurses and other staff can express feelings openly about changes and loss of familiar events and people, such a right is often denied to the people for whom they care. Maureen Oswin (1986), in her research into responses to bereavement and people with mental handicaps, puts forward four possible reasons why staff may be unwilling to speak the truth in circumstances such as these:

1. They may be afraid of losing control of their own emotions in talking about such a sad event.
2. They may be unsure of how they will manage to comfort and control the emotions of the person who is grieving, particularly if they suspect that he might break down in tears or express real anger.
3. They may believe that the bereaved person is like a small child and will not understand such concepts as loss or death, and so feel that it is 'not worth' trying to explain it.
4. They may think that mentally handicapped people do not have the same emotions as people without handicaps, and therefore believe that being told the truth does not matter.

All the above reasons reflect attitudes which may or may not be felt by members of staff. The concept of losing a relationship (for whatever reason) is deemed acceptable for the nurse, but is for some incompatible with personal preconceptions of mental handicap, and certainly not considered to be within the traditional remit of her role.

The nurse and communication skills

It is now accepted that mental handicap nursing skills should be geared towards meeting the needs of the individual client. In order to achieve this, the nurse must possess excellent communication and interpersonal skills. This is recognised by the RNMH 1982 syllabus (see Chapter 1), where communication constitutes one of its nine care concepts. Everyone likes to feel that his or her communication skills are more than adequate. The reality of this may not bear our suppositions out. People with a mental handicap often have problems with communicating. An inability to speak clearly—if at all—will necessitate the use of an alternative form of communication, such as a Blissboard (symbolic representation), or the use of a sign language, such as Makaton.

It is essential, therefore, that the nurse acquire the skills of an effective communicator so that she in turn can enable her client to identify and develop his full potential. Such skills may be acquired through increased self-awareness: 'In listening to what is said, and to what is implicit in what is being said, the nurse can gain new insights through which to modify or develop his or her behaviour' (Burnard, 1985).

The use of such techniques could initially appear time-consuming but in the long term there is much to be gained, with the promise of a more effective outcome for both nurse and client.

The socialisation process

When considering relationships, we should respect the importance of the 'socialisation process'. This process begins within the family unit and later extends out with the family unit as the child starts playgroup or school. Pressures to conform will begin subtly with other children: 'I've got a coat with a blue hood. You haven't!'

The growing child has to cope not only with being away from his family and home environment, but also with trying not to lose face with peers. He learns to play and share with other children. Following the work of developmental psychologists such as Piaget and Bruner, play has been carefully studied and described, resulting in the widely held belief that play '. . . is instrumental for children's mental and emotional growth' (Bruner et al., 1976).

The socialisation process also demands that the individual has beliefs. These may be considered prejudices by some and may be challenged. The accepted role of the adult is to facilitate a learning environment in which the child is able to make sense of and understand his environment more fully. In this way children acquire tolerance by experience and by others' example: 'Children can learn to include the odd one, the handicapped, the slow one. Children can be very generous if this is the way of the playgroup, and as long as they get the necessary support from an adult who will make sure that they are not burdened for too long. This could nurture a quality of compassion in them and make them aware of the needs of others' (Holt and Holt, 1957).

Adolescence brings with it a search for identity, and relationships which were once clearly defined, such as the child–parent relationship, may need to be reassessed and remodelled. As the young person's dependence on his parents lessens, he will become more aware of his individuality and begin to look beyond the family for a sense of identity and belonging. As the individual becomes aware of his physical development, he may recognise his sexuality and begin to feel the need to become sexually active.

As formal education ends, the need to find suitable employment and a sense of self-worth takes on a high priority. External and societal factors affecting employment opportunities and alternatives to them may affect the young person. Occasionally, frustrations and fears fed by lack of motivation among peers, or a high-handed and reproachful attitude on the part of prospective employers combined with a negative attitude generally towards the difficulties experienced by young people, can have a detrimental effect and can lead to symptoms conclusive of what is often labelled as 'delinquency'.

The ability to emerge from this potentially hazardous and traumatic period with a purpose in life and one's dignity intact is crucial to the success or otherwise of the young person's future. 'Conventionally, though not for the people going through them, earlier phases of the life cycle are rather like rehearsals—young people explore, prepare, practise and play with ideas, relationships, jobs and leisure interests' (Rapaport and Rapaport, 1980).

This natural progression through life leads to an established adult in what can potentially be described as the most productive phase of his life.

Failure to form mutually worthwhile relationships, to get and keep a worthwhile job and to continue to see and value a personal purpose in life can lead to feelings of loss or bereavement similar to those discussed earlier. Grief for 'what might have been' can undermine the individual's sense of self-esteem.

The ability to realise and develop our full potential requires those around us to provide the right setting. For those with a mental handicap, the job of providing the right setting is usually left to others, and this in turn can limit the scope and availability of choices for those unable to provide the most appropriate setting for themselves.

Just as every relationship carries with it a chance of being hurt, let down or saddened by another person, so does it carry the chance of great personal happiness. The person with a mental handicap may not be aware of the potential risks involved. Nevertheless, it is his right to be exposed to and experience them, and nurses must recognise and respect this as his need to socialise and integrate with others becomes evident.

Crisis intervention in relationships

The key role of the nurse when a client experiences loss or grief is one of support, particularly where changes in home or life-style become necessary. Supporting and comforting skills are essential prerequisites of the effective nurse, and can be shared and promoted by the entire care team.

Client education

Clients can be helped to experience and cope with relationships. This may be achieved by providing information on such areas as sex, friendships and bereavement, while at the same time showing how such relationships are formed and enjoyed, perhaps using role play and role modelling. Learning to behave appropriately can be a rewarding experience within a peer group which provides a 'safe' setting and approval. Here the individual may start to develop self-awareness and begin to view himself in relation to others: in time he will begin to value his own contribution and attach some worth to himself as a human being.

It is important to realise that the role the nurse plays in developing interpersonal skills will involve teaching others about how to respond positively to their own feelings, fears and inhibitions. In the profiles which follow you will begin to see the profound effects which relationships can have on our lives for good or bad. The reality is that people do not always learn how to cope with the wide range of relationships that they encounter throughout their lives. The opportunity to have a particular relationship may never arise, or specific experiences building up to a relationship may be misunderstood, and so the relationship does not develop.

The loss of a treasured toy to a small child can be a traumatic event for both parents and child, and in later years the loss of a pet or friend can also be quite shattering. The person who does not develop sufficiently to comprehend loss beyond the concept that it is 'gone', no longer to be remembered, is unable to progress satisfactorily towards independent life.

In attempting to cope with the shortfall, the client must have access to all the loving and non-judgemental support that family and carers can muster, so that his emotional equilibrium can be safely restored.

In the following problem, discuss the implications that arise for:

1. Mary.
2. Her parents.
3. Her brother and sister.
4. Residential care staff.

Mary

Mary is a severely mentally handicapped young adult in her early twenties. She lives away from home in a small residential unit. Because of the distance between her family home and the unit, visits from members of the family or a visit home has to be arranged a long time in advance.

Mary moved to residential care in her late teens, as her family, after many long and difficult years, felt this to be the right environment for her. Mary is the youngest of three children. Her sister is married and her

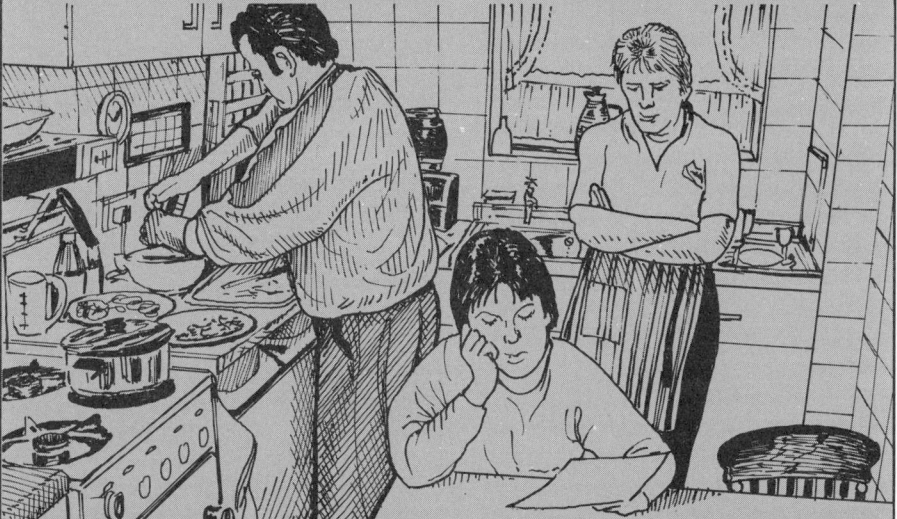

brother lives at home with her parents. Both parents lead active lives, but find caring for Mary on her occasional visits home very demanding and a great strain.

As a child Mary destroyed the contents of the family home. She rarely slept, and when she did, some form of restraint was necessary to prevent injury to herself. Although, in time, the destructive behaviour began to lessen, self-injurious behaviour took a firmer hold. Just as one problem was resolved, so it seemed that another instantly took its place.

The solution arrived at for Mary was residential care. The price to be paid for this, however, was isolation from her family and from her own 'home'. No matter how many times Mary's family visited the unit, no matter how many times she went home on a visit, Mary still grieved to be permanently at home with her family.

When her parents visited and could not take her home with them, Mary's self-injurious behaviour increased and she became very distressed.

When eventually she did go home on a visit, she required constant supervision, as she felt compelled to touch and hold close to her ornaments and other familiar objects in the house. Even when Mary was offered familiar objects or photographs to take back to the unit with her, this failed to satisfy or appease her. Her home, its contents and the presence of her family was what Mary wanted.

Bill and Annie

Meeting at the Adult Training Centre during lunch breaks was not a very auspicious way to start a relationship. Annie (22 years) had never had a steady boyfriend, although Bill (30 years) had in the past had several girl friends.

Bill was only biding time at the Adult Training Centre. He had lost his job with the Parks Department in the Borough Council and was now helping in the horticultural section, growing plants for the Centre's open day. He was hoping to get another job soon—perhaps a packing job with one of the local stores.

Bill wanted to be independent: living with his mother was all right but a place of his own was really the answer. His mother was not sure about his moving, but with a little persuasion he could change her mind.

Annie's circumstances were quite different. She had never been in employment and it was unlikely that she would ever have a job. Annie

Continued

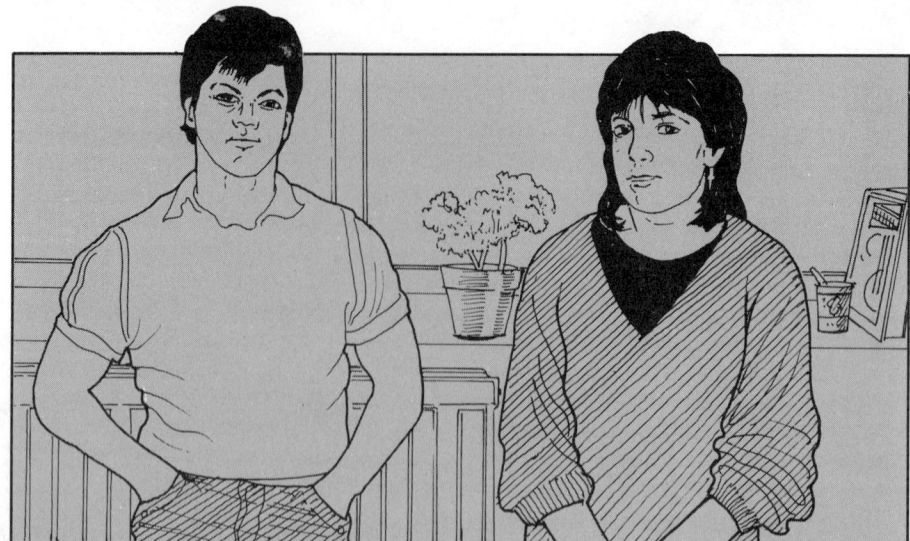

coped well in the home situation, and was able to shop and travel without too much difficulty. From time to time she needed a degree of supervision so that managing her money did not become a problem.

This close supervision was provided by Annie's mother and sisters, with whom she lived. Her mother was a determined woman who often said that her middle daughter (Annie) would always need her and that there was no chance that Annie would ever be able to cope away from home.

Annie's mother disapproves of her daughter's relationship with Bill. She considers him idle and 'up to no good'. She will not allow him into the house, and restricts Annie going out with him by not allowing her to answer the door or telephone.

After about a year Bill proposed to Annie and she accepted. Both mothers were disapproving about the impending marriage. Eventually, with some discussion between the two families, Annie's and Bill's sisters managed to arrange the wedding.

Once married, Annie and Bill lived in a council flat. Annie was still attending the Adult Training Centre and Bill looked for work. Within their first year of marriage, Annie became pregnant. Both of them said they wanted a baby, but Annie's mother seemed convinced that her daughter was open to a degree of sexual harassment and that the pregnancy was a mistake.

Annie's mother began to exclude Bill from her home again. When the couple visited, Annie would be taken upstairs on the pretext of having her hair done and Bill would not see her for the rest of the day. In the end he would leave and go walking the streets until the evening, when he and Annie would return to their home.

Discuss the nurses' responsibility in this situation, and the role of the professionals.

(a) Possible solutions

There is no prescriptive answer to any of the points raised in the above profiles. The initial reaction felt on reading about Mary or Annie and Bill will have much to do with your attitudes as an individual. Perhaps a lack of experience will cause you to feel embarrassed or confused about the questions posed.

In analysing these profiles and future real-life situations, the emphasis should be on responding to a crisis. The mnemonic CRISIS can be a useful *aide-memoire* to help unravel the complex information and detail in a given situation.

CRISIS stands for:

Characters   Who are the main persons involved? What part do they play?
Relationships   What connections exist between the people concerned?
Interferers   Who influences the relationship externally?
Surroundings   What impact does the environment have on the characters and the nature of the relationship?
Indicators   What are the warning signs that highlight the problems?
Solutions   What is your answer and how would you justify it?

Conclusion

This chapter has looked at the enormous topic of relationships. It is based on the assumption that every human being has a right to benefit from personal experience, even though we know that for the person with a mental handicap this right is not always acknowledged.

Remember that '. . . the handicapped have a right to love and be loved and a right to be hurt. This is part of the human condition.' (Greengross, 1976).

References

Bruner, J., Jolly, A. and Sylva, K. (eds), *Play, Its Role in Development and Evolution*, Penguin, 1976

Burnard, P. *Learning Human Skills*, Heinemann, 1985

Copperman, H. *Dying at Home*, Wiley, 1983

Greengross, W., *Entitled to Love*, Malaby Press, London, 1976

Holt, K. and Holt, S., The Influence of a Retarded Child on Family Limitations, *American Journal of Mental Deficiency Research*, **3**, 28–34, 1957

Oswin, M. Bereavement and Mentally Handicapped People, Kings Fund discussion paper, Kings Fund, London, 1986

Rapaport, R. and Rapaport, R. *Growing through Life*, Harper and Row, 1980

Reed, E. W. and Reed, S. C., *Mental Retardation: A Family Story*, Saunders, 1965

Seligman, M. E. P., *Helplessness*, Freeman, 1975

Wolfensburger, W., *Normalisation*, National Institute of Mental Retardation, Toronto, 1972

Further reading

Craft, M., Bicknell, J. and Hollins, S., *Mental Handicap*, Baillière Tindall, 1985

Craft, A. and Craft, M., *Handicapped Married Couples*, Routledge and Kegan Paul, 1979

Craft, A. and Craft, M., *Sex and the Mentally Handicapped*, RKP, 1986

Mattinson, J., *Marriage and Mental Handicap*, 2nd edn, Institution of Marital Studies, Tavistock Institute of Human Relations, London, 1975

Sines, D. and Bicknell, J., *Caring for Mentally Handicapped People in the Community*, Harper and Row, 1985

Whelan, E. and Speake, B., *Learning to Cope*, Souvenir Press, 1979

Chapter 5

Caring in the community
by Gillian James

Introducing the concept of community care

In the past few years the concept of care for people with a mental handicap has been to integrate or keep this specialist group within a community setting. Perhaps the most forward-thinking document of its day, *Better Services for the Mentally Handicapped*, was published in 1971 and set the trends for policy in services up to the end of this century, with a major shift in responsibility involving an increasing need for local provision and requiring a full supporting network.

In the 1970s many reports and a general plethora of information were made available to all interested parties on how these advances could be made, with a wide dissemination of new ideas coming from many sources. Indeed we saw the beginning of a new breed of nurse — the Community Mental Handicap Nurse — evolve.

The pioneers began to go forth into the then unknown field of community mental handicap care, investigating the needs, often in very practical terms, of the families who had maintained a handicapped person within their own home setting, and providing at least some basic resources which parents most desperately needed. The Community Mental Handicap Nurses' role developed, well supported by documentation of some skills acquired in this very new and testing environment.

Numbers of Community Mental Handicap Nurses rose from single figures to over one thousand in a space of a few short years. Such were the changes and advances made that we now have a well-established and rightly recognised group of specialists working with and for families in community settings.

Governments of the day recognised the changing pattern of care developing, as did the nursing profession, both on the management of the services side and on the need for changes in statutory training requirements for nurses working in this field.

A huge shift of emphasis was beginning to become apparent. Professionals and voluntary agencies alike were not satisfied with the many facets of care, training and service patterns, and many wanted change and answers to very searching questions. The media were all too ready to follow up lines of investigation, particularly regarding the care given in the longer-stay institutions. Many hospitals were subject to investigations which highlighted several problems and suggested ways of improvement.

The General Nursing Council for England and Wales reviewed the training syllabus for nurses in the mental handicap field, and in 1982 prepared a brand-new syllabus representing a whole shift of emphasis of care and including, in Section Seventeen, training to facilitate integration and rehabilitation into the community.

The present position of the Community Nurse in Mental Handicap is such that those working in the field are facing a challenge as never before, with new philosophies, new horizons and new opportunities to develop and practise their skills as client needs change. Expectations are often beyond the resources at present available but the Community Nurse in Mental Handicap is ready and willing to face that challenge now.

Community care, philosophy and networking

The philosophy of care as stated in the 1971 *Better Services for the Mentally Handicapped* document is still quoted as the way forward, and is supported by each major document that has been produced since that time. Attendant to the right of each mentally handicapped person to be treated as an individual comes recognition that each requires additional help from the professional services and from the community where he or she lives in order to develop fully as an individual.

This is where the major thrust of community care lies. A fully supportive network of services is recommended, with emphasis on the mentally handicapped person and family receiving support both in practical resource terms and in helping to alleviate the many problems they have to face in the community today.

Planning, developing and reviewing need

When planning a local service, it is important to identify needs and resources and 'match them up' in order to provide a meaningful service to a mentally handicapped person and his family.

It is important to have a joint philosophy which is developed around the need to provide a full range of services in the community, and to include a choice of residential accommodation which is developed around the individual. Families need to have access to these services, which, if reasonably flexible, would allow for anticipated needs as well as the emergencies which will occur from time to time.

A co-ordinated system of care is important, as is an awareness of the direction in which agencies are moving and how resources are being used to develop the service. There should be no wide gaps in the service, and collaboration by professional and voluntary agencies in looking at the total need should avoid this.

The overall implications of keeping a mentally handicapped person in the community, and moving people from hospital into the community, should be planned carefully. Staff should be involved wherever possible, so that a greater commitment to any new proposals is gained and maintained.

Any services planned should be constantly reviewed, as proposals often have to be changed to meet changing resources and need. A proactive service should (where possible) be established with an acceptable community interface.

Teamwork approach

The goal of good teamwork must be to establish and maintain links for people with a mental handicap and their families, to provide specialist help when and where needed, and by improving domiciliary support to enable the family to make a positive contribution to their management, care and training.

In order to realise this goal, there are several aims which would need to be satisfied, as follows:

1. To provide a platform for all agencies to work together.
2. To identify existing resources available.
3. To establish a system of identifying this client group.
4. To bring to the families an awareness of local services and facilities available to them.
5. To act as the first point of contact for the family in order to provide advice and help.
6. To help co-ordinate access to services which have often been seen as fragmented in the past.
7. To prevent hospital admission wherever possible.
8. To seek to provide alternative accommodation as and when required.
9. To provide very specialised help to the family.
10. To help to establish a close working relationship with relevant voluntary organisations and groups.
11. To assist in the relocation of mentally handicapped hospital residents into community settings.

Community Mental Handicap Teams have evolved over the past decade in order to improve domiciliary support and meet the ever-changing needs of people with a mental handicap and their family within a specialist multi-disciplinary framework.

Recently most teams seem to cover population catchment areas of between sixty thousand and eighty thousand people, and have two identified team structures—the Main Group and the Core Teams. The important thing is that they serve the *local community*. In 1986 the 'Community Nursing Review Team for England' specifically identified ways in which neighbourhood networking could be established, but suggested much smaller catchment areas of between ten thousand and twenty-five thousand people.

The community mental handicap team is made up of representatives from those professions and voluntary agencies which are responsible for, or have an interest in, this specialist group. A wide range of specialists may be involved— i.e. National Health Service, social services, special education experts, and parent representatives, who co-operate fully as 'partners' with the professionals.

Many have defined their role within agreed terms of reference. Meetings may range in frequency from weekly for Core Teams, to monthly or quarterly for Main Groups. Accountability often seems to be blurred, but some strongly believe that true accountability should be to clients and families.

It is important that the Main Groups have not only annual goals, but also short-term objectives, the framework existing to bring together all those involved in mental handicap, with a clear focus on providing a comprehensive service network within the local community (see Figure 5.1).

Aims and Objectives

1. Give support to families.
2. Identify existing provisions.
3. Compile and maintain an accurate register of clients.
4. Monitor service provision.
5. Help plan development and organisation of a satisfactory service.
6. Highlight problems/needs.
7. Mobilise resources.
8. Monitor plans.
9. Provide information to specialists and others.
10. Act as adviser to other multidisciplinary teams and specialist groups.
11. Promote the service.
12. Discuss problems.
13. Act as a two-way resource centre.
14. Be a pressure group.
15. Check that reviews and any statutory obligations are met.

Figure 5.1

The chairperson should be elected democratically. When setting aims and objectives, it is important to be realistic and define achievable goals which should take into account resources available and cost effectiveness. However, it is important that any deficiencies in the service be highlighted. New development must be in the best interests of the consumers, who must be adequately represented at all levels.

Community Mental Handicap Team members and, in particular, parent representatives should have access to facilities for training and development— e.g. conferences, seminars, workshops and other organised activities related to the field of mental handicap. Information on these should be made available and attention drawn to them on a regular basis.

To provide a broad knowledge base for the group, others should be invited to participate in meetings: for example, from colleges, health centres, careers advisory services, community health councils, child development centres, community units, home visiting services and community voluntary services. It is only when real partnership is achieved that the service will develop and relationships begin to improve.

(a) Core teams

The Core Team has as its nucleus a community nurse, a specialist social worker and possibly one other member. They should be full-time members of that team and it is helpful if they are all based together for ease of access.

Meeting on a very regular basis, they have specific aims and objectives and are the central point of contact for everyone involved, to ensure that the service reaches the mentally handicapped person and family. They also act as co-ordinators, to allow the family to obtain help when needed and identify the key worker. Core Teams will accept referrals from any source, will decide whether the referral is appropriate and will agree on what action is to be taken.

The Core Team has a responsibility to:
- Deal with problems and enquiries.
- Act as a co-ordinator.
- Share skills by working as a team.
- Plan care.
- Maintain personal files on clients.
- Provide information on latest aids and equipment.
- Check on reviews and case conferences held.
- Check that all needs are attended to and cross-refer as necessary.
- Contribute to discussions on clients' needs.
- Provide colleagues and other appropriate personnel with information from discussions held and keep them informed of any changes.
- Ensure that families are actively involved in any decision-making which directly affects them.
- Hold meetings regularly.
- Transmit information on case transfers or case closures.
- Inform line managers if further resources are required.
- Bring awareness to others of the service and facilities offered and available.
- Support families when problems occur.
- Provide specialist help.
- Support one another.
- Be involved in assisting the placement of hospital residents into community settings.

1 The key worker's (case co-ordinator's) role

The key worker is a named member who will be the main link person with the mentally handicapped person and family. The responsibility of the key worker is to assess, initiate and monitor any planned care and co-ordinate those services offered to the client and family.

The key worker acts as the first point of contact for the family, to provide help, advice and support, having the means to contact other agencies as necessary. The key worker will carry out initial and subsequent assessments, identify problem areas and plan appropriate programmes. He or she must ensure that the plan is carried out and review it as necessary. The key worker will report back to the Core Team and attend all meetings involving the family concerned, thereby ensuring that they are adequately represented at all times.

When appointing the key worker, an important consideration is the effectiveness of the service to the mentally handicapped person. It is essential, therefore, that he or she be chosen with the joint agreement of the Core Team.

The length of the key worker's involvement with the client must be constantly reviewed as circumstances alter. When the problem has been resolved or support from the team is no longer needed, or another key worker is required for a specific reason, then the client's case is reviewed and either discharged from the 'active' list or passed on to the appropriate agency.

2 The role and function of the Community Mental Handicap Nurse

As the role of the Community Mental Handicap Nurse (CMHN) has developed and grown and many of the tasks have now been identified in the systematic approach to planning care, it has naturally increased our professional strength and skills.

Central to the function of the CMHN is the identification of the capabilities of each mentally handicapped person and the planning and implementation of programmes based on his individual needs.

It is important to collect accurate information from the family, and this may include baseline evaluations in the preparation and rolling forward of all individual programmes. The aim must be to raise the level of functioning and enhance the quality of life of both the mentally handicapped person and the family. This may involve improving existing skills, identifying real or potential problems, planning programmes and bringing in other specialist help as and when required; and developing intervention strategies in ways which can be understood by everyone concerned.

Help may be needed to develop early motor, cognitive and self-help skills towards independence, social, interpersonal and decision-making, or help regarding specific sensory and physical disabilities, incontinence, aggressive/destructive behaviour to either self or others, disturbed behaviour, over-activity, noisiness, excessive attention-seeking or persistent wandering.

Much of the CMHN's time will be spent in giving specific help and advice to parents. The provision of practical help, support and advice to parents on the management of the mentally handicapped person is vital. The CMHN needs to recognise any difficulties the family may have *before* they reach crisis point. She must identify the problem areas and help the family, supporting decisions made in the best interests of the mentally handicapped person at that time.

Parents may need advice on lifting techniques, help with managing any dietary requirements and associated problems, and guidance on problems associated with other specific disabilities such as epilepsy or spasticity.

Parents will need to know about the benefits of correct posture, adequate exercise and sleep for their child, and how to recognise and cope with ill-health. They will need advice on aspects of child development and about the allowances and benefits system. Parents will need support and help through natural anxieties about their child's progress in development, education and training, and in coping with the major transitions through life.

CMHNs will need to develop further the skills that parents have to enable them to carry out programmes in the absence of professionals.

Families will sometimes go through stages of retaliation, isolation and withdrawal, and it is important that the nurse identify and understand this and adapt coping skills accordingly.

CMHNs often feel that they are in a good position to extend their role and act as their clients' advocates. By informing and supporting the mentally handicapped person and the family on a variety of issues and situations, the advocate may improve the pattern of their lives considerably.

Advocacy can be carried out in areas such as:

1 Providing information on rights.
2 Supporting their needs as a family.
3 Explaining the role of statutory bodies.
4 Explaining statutory obligations.
5 Helping the mentally handicapped person and/or the family reach decisions.
6 Providing support at interviews and in official settings.
7 Acting as confidante in the family.

It is possible to develop self-advocacy in this field, and every opportunity should be given to the person with a mental handicap to attain this skill and be given support as necessary. The CMHN may also wish to set up and run activity groups for parents and people with a mental handicap, and this should be encouraged.

The aim to maintain the person with a mental handicap in a community setting should always be central to the nurse's task. Care must be taken to meet these needs and not allow interagency problems to be seen as more important than the mentally handicapped person himself. The RCN role document will give further guidance.

Community resources

There are a number of resources which are available to the CMHN, which, if used skillfully, will enhance the service and provide information of benefit to both nurses and families.

Local facilities should provide for a wide range of alternatives for parents' use, and may include local support networks, family support groups, sitting-in services, toy libraries, short-stay facilities, holiday play-schemes, youth club activities, advice and information centres, and shared care schemes. Community experience in working with people with a mental handicap can be gained by schools, Scout and Guide movements, Air Training Corps, Sea Cadets and many other voluntary services, and these should be encouraged and developed.

Nationally there are a variety of very specialist organisations providing up-to-date information on mental handicap care. These include the Royal Society for Mentally Handicapped Children and Adults (MENCAP), the British Institute of Mental Handicap, the Association of Professions for Mentally Handicapped People, the Spastics Society and the Royal College of Nursing Society of Mental Handicap Nursing.

Confidentiality

One of the areas which must be highlighted is that of confidentiality of information involving the mentally handicapped person and his family and third parties who have access to information about that family.

Regard for confidentiality should not be underestimated, and great care and thought should be given to ensure that strict confidentiality is maintained.

When considering confidentiality, the following guidelines should be examined:

1. *DHSS 1985 Code on Confidentiality of Personal Health Information.*
2. *H.C. (84) 10 DHSS Steering Group on Health Services Information (Körner Report).*
3. *The Data Protection Act 1984*, which regulates the use of automatically processed information relating to individuals.

When interviewing families, and assessing and recording information about them, respect for that client and family must be paramount and great care must be taken to ensure that such information remains confidential.

When arranging methods of storing and using information, clear guidelines need to be met and the following questions asked:

- Is the recording manual?
- Is it automatically processed?
- Who has access to the information?
- Is the access to part of or all of the information in the personal file?
- Who gives this permission?
- When recorded, what further use is made of the information?
- Will the clients/families have access to their own personal health information?
- Does a multidisciplinary ethics committee exist which may be referred to in the district?

Community structure and models of care

In examining the community structure, we need to look at the changing pattern of society itself. The stereotyped image of society has dramatically changed, and awareness of individuality and the opportunity to experiment have led to more flexibility in the eyes of the general public. Through lack of understanding resulting from historical segregation and institutionalisation, people with a mental handicap have had a negative image and low social status in the past. However, acceptance by the community is improving. There are still a great many issues to be overcome, and attitudinal change will probably only improve with the education of the population as a whole.

The principle of developing, for people with a mental handicap, independence which is acceptable to others and age-appropriate is widely accepted, and opportunities to integrate them into the community within normal social groups are increasing rapidly. However, any new service has to be demonstrably better, and provide a full range of opportunities in education, employment, places to live, social recreation and leisure, and meeting and mixing with fellow citizens.

Most health districts in England have developed local strategies for mental handicap services, and indeed Wales has developed a National All Wales Strategy. Planning is done within agreed catchment areas, with professionals and interested bodies working closely together with the aim of providing an effective and efficient service.

Planning and management of community mental handicap services

When organising and maintaining community services for people with mental handicap and their families, it is important that the services provided adequately reflect the needs of the defined catchment area.

Community care must essentially provide an adequate support network which is complementary to all other services provided in that area. It must be appropriate for the consumers and be a part of the total and supportive to, rather than a substitute for, other locally based services for people with mental handicap. In order to facilitate the functioning of an adequate community service, options should be examined and, if necessary, existing patterns of service investigated and new proposals organised to reflect the needs of the individual wherever possible. No attempt should be made to introduce a model of care and then try to fit the prospective customers around that service!

It is, therefore, absolutely essential that any planning, implementation and evaluation of community mental handicap services reflect this. Planners should be in a position to facilitate the implementation of proposed structures. Those who are going to receive the service must be well represented, as their priorities and options may well be totally different from those highlighted by the planners. A wide range of services should be made available, to meet the varying needs of this specialist group, such as providing preventive and early intervention, advisory counselling services and responsible management of service delivery. Mental handicap care should not be seen as isolated from the rest of community services; rather it should be seen as part of the total and as encouraging a healthy relationship between the specialists and other professional or voluntary groups.

So that planners have insight into the development of existing services and show how this is perceived, those responsible for service management must be closely involved with what is proposed. Any plans must be consistent with the overall philosophy and have clear and carefully defined objectives.

Those involved in the proposals should make sure that when actual buildings and services are introduced, those interpreting them should know exactly what the proposals really involve.

Resource implications are always an important factor but should not totally dominate any decisions made. Equally important is that planners should not try to implement a model of service into an area if it is not appropriate or if it has serious delaying factors in the development of that service.

When looking at overall community services, planners must satisfy themselves that the range of services proposed dovetails into other existing or proposed plans, fulfils any statutory duties and provides a totally adequate service. Planners must take into account both national and regional policies and guidelines, as well as local needs and set priorities.

Knowledge of the local area is essential. Trends, local and national, sociological and demographic, must be taken into account, staffing being a very important consideration. Multidisciplinary participation should be used positively and effectively. Staff should be encouraged and motivated in order to gain fulfilment from their contribution.

Individual management styles should be allowed to develop within the framework of service delivery. Ongoing service developments should be continually monitored and evaluated, to ensure that acceptable standards are maintained.

Managers are the key advisers in forward planning budgeting, estimating projected needs and investing in future service by good utilisation of staff, and in providing professional support so that a first class service is a reality rather than an ideal.

References

DHSS, *The Community Nursing Review Team Report for England* (Cumberlege), 1986

English and Welsh National Boards for Nursing, Midwifery and Health Visiting Syllabus of Training: Professional Register—Part 5 (Registered Nurse for the Mentally Handicapped), 1982

HMSO, *Better Services for the Mentally Handicapped*, Cmnd 4683, 1971

Royal College of Nursing, Society of Mental Handicap Nursing, *The Role and Function of the Domiciliary Community Nurse for People with a Mental Handicap*, 1985

Further reading

British Institute of Mental Handicap, *Community Mental Handicap Teams: Theory and Practice*, 1986

Brunel Institute of Organisation and Social Studies, *Organisation of Multi-disciplinary Community Teams*, John Øvretveit, 1986

DHSS, *Mental Handicap 'Progress, Problems and Priorities'*, (a review of Mental Handicap Services in England since the 1971 White Paper), 1980

DHSS, *Care in the Community* (a consultative document on moving resources for care in England), 1981

HMSO, House of Commons Social Services Committee Session 1984–85. *Community Care with Special Reference to Adult Mentally Ill and Mentally Handicapped*, Vol. 1: Part VII, The Wider Community, pp. 129–131; Part VIII, 'Clients and Families, pp. 148–151, 'Community Mental Handicap Nurses', pp. 197–198

Royal College of Nursing, Society of Mental Handicap Nursing, *Assuring Quality in the Private Sector: Residential Services in the Community for People with a Mental Handicap*, 1987

United Kingdom Central Council for Nursing, Midwifery and Health Visiting, Project 2000, 'A New Preparation for Practice', 1986

Chapter 6

Alternatives to community care
by Mary Birchenall

The nurse and self-awareness

It may seem strange to begin considering the care of others through looking at one's self, but knowledge of self is an essential prerequisite for establishing a positive caring practice.

An easy beginning in self-examination is to investigate personal reasons for undertaking the care of others. There are no right and wrong answers, only explanations which you can use to create positive care patterns. Few people have 'bad' reasons for caring for others; in turn, a realistic examination of personal motives will help all carers to realise that caring is a two-way interaction, a partnership between themselves and those in their care which is influenced as much by the carer's personal characteristics as by the personality and handicap of those for whom they care. As the discussion on residential care unfolds, it will become clear that to encourage genuine independence to some degree for even the most handicapped person requires the carer to move beyond 'looking after' someone. It is necessary to seek a deeper meaning of 'caring' which includes a possible redundancy for the carer in all or some Activities of Daily Living (see Figure 6.1).

The phrase 'residential care' in this chapter incorporates all care bases, from the foster-home to the hospital ward. Wherever care takes place and whoever provides that care, certain desirable qualities must ideally exist.

The essential requirements of good care practice stem from a basis that care is provided for the benefit of those in receipt of care. Although we may be tempted to take this for granted, experience shows that organisational and personal motives must be recognised as such and not be confused with the care needs of the individual (Goffman, 1974).

For example, if an organisation demands efficiency and busy workers, then the care provided will be organisation-based rather than client-based. Being able to recognise the constraints of both personal and system demands help us to embark on a more positive and individualised care plan.

The basis for all care should be a sound knowledge, based on a nationally recognised professional education or training for anyone who is looking after someone who is not a relative. In the absence of such training, the carer should seek out such resources as the new Open University package, which can be undertaken at home. This package will also enhance the knowledge of any 'qualified' carer.

Basic skill requirements

The basic skills required by the carer include creating opportunities for the development of individual potential in life and social skills attainment: personal development which includes acquiring the necessary self-respect, self-motivation, and an appreciation of the value and dignity of other people.

Until now this chapter has avoided the term 'mental handicap', taking the view that caring for people has many generic components. For example, the need to be self-aware and conscious of organisational constraints is relevant in all areas of care, as are the skill requirements listed above. The intention of omitting the phrase 'mental handicap' until this point is to emphasise that the premise of this text is firmly based on 'normalisation'. Care is seen to promote life chances through stimulating personal development. The roots of care for mentally handicapped people must lie within the framework of 'normality', specialist knowledge being directed towards the achievement of goals which may appear impossible at first within the person's immediate environment.

This section and those following will use that specialist knowledge to provide insights and information about precipitating the growth of the individual who has a mental handicap.

(a) Life and social skills

The categories for life and social skills which will feature in this text have been suggested by Roper, Logan and Tierney, in their Model of Nursing, 'The Activities of Daily Living'. They identify twelve Activities of Living which form a useful guide to basic living skills. These are:

- Maintaining a safe environment.
- Breathing.
- Eliminating.
- Controlling body temperature.
- Working and playing.
- Sleeping.
- Communicating.
- Eating and Drinking.
- Personal cleansing/dressing.
- Mobilising.
- Expressing sexuality.
- Dying.

In their text Roper *et al.* give examples of ways to use their Model of Nursing and examples of the type of paperwork they have devised. Figure 6.1 provides an initial assessment of a profoundly mentally handicapped young man, using the Activities of Daily Living. It is a brief account and *does not* provide a care plan. It does elaborate on ways of interpreting the activities of living, which makes them relevant to mental handicap. A good exercise would be to devise a care plan which would guide his carers in developing his full potential.

1 Preparing written care plans

There is some criticism of using a standardised format such as the Activities of Living form to create an individualised care programme. A major concern is that filling in forms can be time-consuming and detract from face-to-face care. Forms by their nature can create a restrictive pattern which encourages unnecessary replication of information throughout the ward or home, so reducing the level of individualised care and establishing an institutional format. But set against this is the need for care staff to have a common record of care for each individual which can be referred to as necessary by a new team member or a relief nurse. Care plans can also help when explaining future plans to the resident and his relatives, and provide a continuous reference for case reviews. Subsequently, the use of a package, such as one of the various 'Models of Care', which is based on a sound theoretical formulation is advocated for all nurses. Such models are versatile and can be applied in any care setting. Various models have become established as a result of the moves towards holistic nursing care, where the emphasis is placed on the patient as a person with complex needs beyond any specific condition precipitating admission to hospital.

It is the need to have a unified workforce which creates the need to have written care plans. The nurse who works shifts and is a member of a team needs a concrete base to work from. The assessment sheet in Figure 6.1 ensures that all the nurses who come into contact with this young man work towards shared goals, based on a common core of information.

2 Involvement of clients in planning care

An important part of writing a care plan is to involve the mentally handicapped person in the planning. Those who are moderately handicapped can take a direct part in deciding which skills to work towards and the nature of the path they wish to follow. It is likely that they will need a great deal of guidance in the beginning, which should be slowly reduced as they develop decision-making skills. The more profoundly handicapped person, with limited understanding of the reasoning behind and benefits of working towards self-help and socially mature behaviour, can still offer positive input in the creation of his personal care plan, even if unable to use conventional language.

It is the nature of the nurse's role to make observations of the individual which lead to an awareness of those aspects of his life-style which give pleasure and of those which may limit his progress towards acceptable adult patterns of behaviour. In this way the nurse can devise a care plan which is tailored to the individual needs of the resident, taking account of his personal preferences. For example, it is usual to stimulate desired responses by giving rewards. To create an individualised care plan, it is essential to know what would be considered a reward by that resident, rather than to give a standardised 'nice' thing, such as sweets. If you return to thinking about yourself and conjure up a personal list of rewards, you will find that it is both long and diverse. The same should be true for any resident in your care.

The emphasis in mental handicap care is at present directed towards working from the strengths of the individual. This is considered to be more positive than the traditional problem-solving approach. It is proposed here that nursing models offer a framework which combines the positive aspects of both the 'strengths' and the 'problem-solving' approaches. Through combining these ideological stances, an immediate advance is made towards working within the 'normalisation' principle.

1. Activity of Living	2. Usual routines/ what can, cannot be done independently	3. Patient's problems (actual and potential)	4. Goals	5. Nursing interventions	6. Evaluation/ outcome
Eating and drinking	Can drink unaided but quickly. Uses knife and fork but has a tendency to choke on too large pieces of food. Has a healthy appetite but is unable to recognise when he is 'full'; can continue to eat until he vomits, causing upset to client, staff and others at the table.	Actual problems with knowing when to stop eating. Possibility of choking or inhaling vomit. Mealtimes very stressful.	To teach proper use of utensils; to encourage good table manners; to help the patient to recognise when a sufficient amount of food has been consumed. To reduce risk of vomiting and minimise danger of choking and inhalation of vomit. To maintain a balanced diet with appropriate amount of fluids and fibre. To make mealtimes more relaxed and sociable occasions.	To assist with use of knife and fork—i.e. to teach by example. Supervision of mealtimes in as reassuring and relaxed a way as possible, making sure that the client is never left alone. Danger of choking minimised by providing small portions at a time and teaching the client to cut and tear food properly and to eat more slowly. Swallowing techniques are explained each mealtime and the client is praised and encouraged for each achievement, however small.	Client now takes more time over drinking, but still requires a great deal of help and supervision with cutting and swallowing food. Mealtimes now slightly more relaxed but persistence required. The presence of a nurse at the dinner table appears to reassure the client and other diners and improve the general atmosphere. Choice of food could be improved and served in smaller quantities more often rather than in one large meal.
Eliminating	Has a tendency to diarrhoea. Toilet training is partly successful, but he has a tendency to attract attention to himself by soiling and becoming incontinent during the day. Is occasionally incontinent on waking.	Potential soreness of skin and breakdown of skin due to moisture and irritation. Client needs to find a way of attracting attention to himself in a more acceptable and dignified way. His personal morale is in danger of being lowered as a result of poor toilet habits.	To promote continence and to encourage a sense of personal pride and dignity in establishing and maintaining good toilet habits. To prevent skin soreness and encourage personal cleanliness. To eliminate incontinence on wakening where possible.	Special attention is given to the client every time he behaves in a socially acceptable manner. Client is involved in decision-making and discussion to reduce feelings of isolation. Client is taught basic skin care and praised for dryness and requests to go to the toilet. He is encouraged to carry out his personal hygiene himself with adequate time and privacy allowed.	Client is still incontinent on waking, but a gentle reminder about 7 a.m. occasionally works. Skin condition is much improved, but should be checked regularly in a discreet way.

Figure 6.1 Patient assessment form

Each human individual has both strengths and weaknesses, complementary and problematic traits, which intermix to create the complex persona he presents to the world. In the same way the mentally handicapped person experiences a complex mixture of strengths, weaknesses and problems. As can be seen in the brief example given, both strengths and weaknesses are highlighted. In this way, new skills to be achieved can be based on the successes of past learning; also, the degree of deficit or competence is clearly indicated.

The nurse learns that although the patient in the example is continent, he has further achievements to make before he has mastered this skill. She may consider finding a more positive bargaining counter, and establish a reason for being continent. The positive aspects of continence may seem obvious to the average person, but without the social reinforcement which provides us with reasons for maintaining a continent manner, there is no real reason for continence. We shall consider this in more detail as we take up the concepts of 'dignity' and 'self-respect'.

The activity 'Eliminating' was deliberately chosen in the example as it directs us towards a consideration of the concepts of dignity, self-motivation, self-respect and valuing others. If the reader should choose to create a mental picture of a dignified man, it is reasonable to assume that a taken-for-granted characteristic would be continence. That is, it would be unthinkable that overt incontinence and dignity should travel together. As a society we place so much importance on continence that the majority of mothers are looking for toilet training in their infants to be completed by the end of the second year of life. Playgroups and nurseries can and do require children to be toilet-trained. It is hardly exceptional, then, that care establishments, and perhaps nurses in particular, seem obsessed with toilet training. Advocacy Alliance, in their booklet, consider the setting up of toilet training programmes for residents in long-stay hospitals a measure of their success. The achievement of continence is a socially important skill, related to the value society places upon a person, and is viewed as a measure of maturity. To be obviously incontinent, wearing incontinence pads or being escorted as an adult to the toilet can influence the growth of self-respect and dignity.

This does not imply that the incontinent person must remain undignified, but it does mean that the nurse must be very aware of her personal feelings about incontinence. Each nurse carries with her social attitudes developed over the years of her childhood and early adult life. These attitudes are so much part of her that she is largely unaware that she holds them. The nurse who consciously or unconsciously abhors dealing with faeces, smeared bodies and clothing, but suppresses her feelings 'to get the job done', can signal to the resident feelings which express her disgust and thus give the impression that their relationship in some way demeans her.

In such an instance dignity would be slow in developing, despite outward techniques being exemplary, and the nurse would remain unaware of her unconsciously imposed limitations. This returns us to the need to be 'self-aware': any aspect of care which offends or hurts the nurse requires careful self-examination. The ideal work situation should encourage open discussion of such problems.

It is important for the nurse to realise that disliking certain aspects of her work need not influence her relationship with the resident in a detrimental way, nor should it be seen as a personal failure.

Care of the profoundly handicapped person

The resident who is both profoundly mentally handicapped and physically disabled requires total nursing care. Many of the twelve activities of daily living will occur only through the assistance and intervention of the nurse, such as eating, dressing and communicating. Often, time given to carrying out this care can occupy the nurse to such an extent that there is little time to reflect on the *quality* of that care. Some hospital wards can have a staff : patient ratio as high as 1 : 6. Subsequently, the demands of providing a high quality of physical care can overwhelm the nurse, and leave her too exhausted to think about extending that good practical care towards stimulating a growth of independence.

To some it may seem incongruous to consider development and independence in a discussion of severe physical and mental handicap. The combination of such severe disabilities can overwhelm the senses and convince the nurse that she is right to provide absolute and total care, making all necessary decisions on behalf of the resident.

This would seem to imply that character, determination and the ability to indicate personal preference are not part of the make-up of the profoundly handicapped person — a statement which we know to be categorically untrue! Experience has shown that even the most profoundly handicapped person can and does make progress. The problem seems to be to find some way of combining the daily work load of the care setting with the need to take account of the idiosyncrasies of each individual. To any hard-pressed ward staff this is a tall order.

To discuss a solution, we return to the care plan. Insightful use of the assessment sheets and care plans can guide nurses and highlight those aspects of individuality which the nurse needs to be aware of, during those demanding and busy times which are a regular feature of our timetabled society. These busy periods can monopolise the nurse to the extent that she can overlook the fact that, what for her is a routine and repetitive work process, is, for the resident, fresh each time.

Identifying and stimulating the individuality of the severely handicapped person requires great skill. Nurses in any care establishment need to amass personal knowledge concerning each resident, with detail similar to that of a parent.

Intelligent use of a nursing model can achieve the latter; the written framework will facilitate continuity of care despite shift changes and staff movement. In this way knowledge of everyday things such as which part of a room a resident prefers to sit in need never be lost. This is most important in the formal care context in which there is more than one carer, sharing 24 hour care.

For many nurses with responsibility for several multiply handicapped residents at one time, it can seem an impossible task to give attention and stimulus as well as good basic care. To find a possible solution to this dilemma, we turn to Nicola Schaeffer's work describing her daily care of her multiply handicapped daughter. A particularly interesting discussion in this book is concerned with the idea of people having 'switched-on' and 'switched-off' periods. If learning and communication was to occur in an effective manner, Ms Schaeffer felt she had to be aware of the 'switched-on' moments in her daughter. Similarly, the nurse must become aware of such changes in her clients. The nurse is at risk of becoming defeated by the immensity of the task of caring for the physical, emotional, intellectual and spiritual needs of those in her care, but by developing an awareness of those optimum moments for each resident, some pathway through these seemingly impossible demands can be glimpsed. In the first instance, the nurse must use the 'switched-on' periods to enhance the care she gives. It is unlikely that all residents will be 'switched on' at the same time, and so the task of stimulation becomes achievable even in the busiest of establishments.

Some self-reflection will establish that each individual has peaks and troughs in performance which are reflected in personal results. The handicapped person is no different in this respect, and the nurse should learn that those in her care have good and bad days, too. Care should centre on the individual, rather than timetabled activities organised around the nursing duty rota or institutional management mechanisms.

The more disabled an individual is, the greater the temptation to care for him completely. The nurse must give that person time to become involved in the decisions she makes for him, and so encourage growth. Activities are slower for the multiply handicapped person, and the nurse who feels constrained by time and duty could be trapped into working at her pace rather than the resident's. In this way those precious 'switched-on' moments could be overlooked, yet the physical care be excellent.

Despite the need to perform or assist in every function of daily living, it is unkind and unprofessional to overlook the decision-making potential of the multiply handicapped person. The nurse must be aware of the response of the resident to *all* stimuli.

For example, a common occurrence is to present ready-prepared meals to the resident. 'After all, he has been known to eat anything he was given' has been heard said many times. Yet an observant nurse will note that the resident has definite preferences. He may be unable to make verbal statements, but his responses can be interpreted as positive and enthusiastic or negative and disinterested. The thrill of achievement is also evident; therefore, the nurse should be aware of the small achievements that can be made by the resident. To do otherwise is to deny the resident the possibility of developing skills for himself. For example, it may be quicker to put someone's arm straight into a jumper, but if the resident has the physical ability to push his arm in for himself, then time should be given for this to take place. It may mean finding incentives for this to occur.

Conquering a physical handicap requires a great deal of encouragement. It is unlikely that the profoundly handicapped resident will insist on his right to learn, especially if everything has been done for him for a number of years. Incentives need not be difficult to find: the extra attention and warmth of the nurse's reaction to his initial attempts may be enough in themselves. One thing is certain, however: any sign of impatience on the part of the nurse will act as a disincentive, and the resident will avoid and resist that procedure as a result. It is an unfortunate human trait that discouragement often seems easier to find than encouragement.

Care of the moderately mentally handicapped person

A moderate mental handicap can be a matter for personal interpretation modified by such external factors as measured intelligence (IQ) and the ability to speak and to mobilise. For the purposes of this text, the term 'moderate' refers to people who have some speech, are ambulant and can learn rote tasks. Their measured IQ is not taken into account, since this can inhibit the nurse's awareness of the ability of low-scoring individuals to provide self-care.

It is important on behalf of each individual resident to establish the nature of the help required in achieving each step towards independence. There are many learning processes necessary to move from the 'hotel-style' life of the home or ward towards complete or partial personal care. For the nurse, using the appropriate nursing model will help to highlight strengths and weaknesses in the resident's knowledge and skills. An example of a brief assessment using Orem's Nursing Model is provided in Figure 6.2. This model does not have standardised paperwork, but guides the user to ask set questions which highlight pertinent needs. The reader may like to consider developing a care plan using this brief assessment.

Figure 6.2 **Orem's self-care model**

First Stage
Is there a deficit between the individual's self-care abilities and the demands for self-care?
John has the potential for self-care but 20 years of total care provision in a 'safe' environment has eroded his opportunities to develop and express his skills.

Second Stage
Why is there a self-care deficit?

1. Lack of knowledge?

John has minimal knowledge of how food appears on the table, how clothes become dirty and then clean. His skills for personal care are related to routine such as bath nights rather than being knowledge-based. The detailed skills such as nail care and foreseeing personal needs are outside his present field of control.

2. Lack of skill?

John can dress, bath, feed and toilet himself, choosing clothing appropriate to the occasion and season. He has basic cooking skills if supervised and guided. His decision-making ability is extremely limited. He has good use of English and can make himself understood to strangers. He is hesitant to ask for help from those he does not know.

Continued

3. Lack of motivation?

After 20 years of living on a ward where everything has been done for him, he is having difficulty in coming to terms with self-care. He does want to live in an ordinary house with his two friends, but would prefer other people to do the work. He has difficulty accepting that after a day at work he must return home and cook his own meals etc.

4. Limited range of behaviour?

His life experiences over the past 20 years have emphasised a passive role. His peer group have reinforced this dependent role, being themselves dependent on others. John has subsequently become stereotyped in his behaviour, to the extent of becoming rigid. He is extremely anxious about all aspects of self-care, and when expected to contribute to decision-making or problem-solving sessions, he will withdraw from the situation. If he is unable to withdraw, he becomes apprehensive and can become physically aggressive as a means of coping with this stress.

It is important to avoid overloading the resident when there is a seemingly endless number of skills to be absorbed. If an individual has been looked after, either at home or in care, then it is likely that he will lack many of the skills which the average person takes for granted. Subsequently, the need to practise and master an extensive list can be so daunting as to discourage the resident from the outset.

The nurse must emphasise in her preparatory work those skills already evident. A common occurrence at this point is to emphasise the learning of basic, concrete skills, such as cooking, cleaning, shopping, as being areas of deficit. Indeed, for someone who has no knowledge of how a tin is opened, then providing Sunday dinner will be an enormous task.

Such skills can be and have been achieved successfully, the nurse being able to use a variety of tools from educational and psychological sources. Here we shall consider some less obvious skills in daily living, such as decision-making, self-control, and motivation. The reason for this is linked to the idea of care and control which has been touched on previously. The nurse is held responsible for the quality of care she provides and is therefore conscious of the presentation of the resident to the social world. One result of this is that the nurse ensures that all the basic necessities for living function smoothly and to a high standard. She inadvertently 'takes control', organising the resident's day, perhaps applying artificial standards to his activities. The consequences of the nurse's self-protective strategy are that the resident develops specific skills but remains dependent on those 'in charge' to provide the motivation and to make decisions.

The nurse must be prepared to work at a slower pace, to allow the resident to achieve progress, and to accept less demanding standards than those she traditionally sets. This is not to suggest that the mentally handicapped person will provide himself with substandard care, but rather it is intended to highlight the fact that the nurse, in her working capacity, demands higher standards than she requires of herself at home.

Personal care standards vary from person to person, and it would seem preferable to assist someone to achieve a standard within definable, yet acceptable, limits, rather than emphasise disability by creating conformity. The creation of absolute conformity was never the intention of 'normalisation'. It is a requirement within the theoretical formulations of the 'normalisation' principle that the individual should *live with his handicap*, experiencing as much of everyday living as possible.

An important part of being in control of our everyday lives is the ability to make decisions about both important and small things. Decision-making must feature as a skill to be learned for those with a mental handicap, alongside the more obvious skills such as cooking. If a resident has always had food provided at set times throughout the day, then he may have internalised the knowledge that 'someone always provides'. It is necessary for the resident to learn that there are consequences for himself if he does not provide his own meals, or live within the socially acceptable limits of his chosen community. The nurse must facilitate the resident's learning of two major cognitive steps: *one*, decision making; and *two*, self-responsibility.

Cognitive skills are difficult for the mentally handicapped person to learn and for the nurse to assess. It is essential that control over styles of living be placed in the hands of the resident himself. This may mean that should he decide to avoid preparing his own meal in the hope that someone else will, then he should do without that meal to realise the consequences of disowning his responsibilities towards himself. This may be a contentious statement, especially within the hospital setting, where there could be legal consequences for the carer. In turn, if the care plan is developed with the resident, then the nurse has the opportunity to discuss and explain the details necessary to achieve self-care. The resident is then in a position to agree to experiencing the consequences of his own behaviour.

Realising the consequences of particular experiences is an important part of personal development, and there seems no sound reason for denying this experience to the mentally handicapped individual. If we do, then we are returning to a state of knowledge which was once ruled by the needs of the hospital—to maintain a safe environment at all costs, despite the negative effect this had on development. Not only must the routine process of a task be learned, but also the need for the task and its importance in the resident's life-plan must be made clear to him. In this way the resident begins to take responsibility for himself.

The move towards independence

The progress from adolescent to adult remains a mystery, but it is a clear example of the traumas involved for carers, in 'letting go' and learning the arts of independence. This period of learning is well known for its tempestuous nature as both parties adjust to their new 'roles'. There are parallels here for those with a moderate mental handicap learning to care for themselves. The important lesson for the nurse is that, like the parent, the measure of success is in being able to 'let go', and to cease being needed in an infantile way. Finally, the concept of 'normalisation' has encouraged much thought on creating a sense of value for mentally handicapped people. Creating opportunities for independence and self-help will encourage the resident to value himself and so assist him to act with dignity.

Generating an image that is centred on the mentally handicapped person's abilities rather than disabilities will assist greatly in creating a valued place for mentally handicapped people in our society. Secondary to balancing the public image of mental handicap is the need for the resident to value others. When an individual has a great many demands placed upon him, which he is exhorted to achieve, and is highly praised when he does so, it is almost inevitable that the self becomes dominant.

To consolidate the move towards genuine adulthood and a sense of independence, the resident must be helped to understand that his responsibilities to himself also extend towards others. Through sharing the planning of care between nurse and resident, the first lesson in appreciating and considering others is subconsciously learned. The nurse's personal example of care towards herself and others should provide a model which exemplifies selflessness rather than selfishness. In the same way, the nurse's model of respect for others and for herself should provide a positive model of the way to treat other people.

Worthwhile aims

The basic advice to the nurse in this chapter is to examine the care she gives. First, assess the balance of residents' and organisational needs which dictate the daily routine. Second, observe yourself in your care environment and determine who controls the face-to-face interaction. Third, examine the rule base of your care establishment. Everyone in our society lives by rules. Within our personal living areas, the majority of rules for adults are agreed on a mutual basis. Much effort is needed to ensure that rule-making is shared in residential care. There is a real danger that an efficiently run organisation will exert control over all members in a restrictive manner.

The provision of individualised care is rarely efficient, although always effective, and can seem untidy even in the smallest of community homes. A pertinent reminder of the influence caring individuals have over the achievement of those in care is the example of cerebral palsy. The combination of an inability to communicate, severe physical handicap and the limited expectations of their carer could create a picture of total inability. Today many people with cerebral palsy graduate from university with higher degrees. While persons with a genuine mental handicap may not aspire to educational achievement, those areas that can be attained must not be limited by those who care for them. The nurse who cares for any person with a disability must have as her goal *their achievements* rather than her own.

Further reading

Advocacy Alliance, *Guidelines for One-to-one Advocacy in Mental Handicap Hospitals*, published by themselves, 1984

Aggleton, P. and Chalmers, H., *Nursing Models and the Nursing Process,* Nursing Times and Macmillan Education, 1986

Goffman, E., *Asylums*, Penguin, 1974

Mental Handicap: Patterns for Living, Open University, p. 555, 1986

Schaeffer, N., *Does She Know She's There?*, Harper and Row, 1978

Chapter 7

The nurse as teacher and therapist

by Pat Brudenell

The nurse as educator

(a) What is education?

Education is many things to many people. Unfortunately, many people believe that education for mentally handicapped people is something very specialised, belonging to Special Schools, and more recently to Colleges of Further Education: in effect, that 'special education is special'. Nothing could be further from the truth. Teachers don't have the monopoly on the educational process. If we are working in the field of mental handicap, then we are all in the business of teaching—irrespective of status or discipline.

Before I begin to discuss the role of the nurse as educator, I feel that it is important to establish just what it is we mean by 'education'. I should like to use my favourite definition as the base for this chapter:

Education is a journey of discovery, exploration, growth and development—a widening of horizons and experiences.

If we can agree that education is a life-long process, then we are, in effect, saying that it does not occur at set times of the day with set people. Education is not only life-long; it is also day-long. Education is not Monday to Friday; it is weekends too. Education does not stop for holidays, nor is it simply something which takes place through school years in a designated educational environment. Education is much wider than that. With each day we are faced with new encounters and new experiences. We consolidate these new aspects, within the framework of past and previous experiences, and utilise the new information for future transactions.

This educational process does not start when we go to school and come to a halt when we leave. The process continues throughout our lives.

(b) How do we learn?

We can make a start by looking at some of the elements and people involved in our own learning processes. We learn from parents, peers, relatives, friends, the media, daily interaction, and so on. We learn by listening, watching, tasting, smelling and touching. We learn by design and by accident. We learn through play, exploration and creativity. We cannot say that everything learned has been directly attributable to our attendance at school. And we most certainly cannot say that our learning stopped when we reached a certain age. I believe that people will only learn when, and if, they are ready to do so. It is the relationship between teacher and learner that will determine whether learning will take place. When this relationship is established, learning becomes a two-way process—each party having something to contribute to the other. For the nurse, and in fact for any practitioner, it simply is not enough to acquire the skills to teach. The essence of teaching lies within the recognition, acknowledgement and trust of the relationship that develops between teacher and learner.

Acknowledging the pattern set for ourselves, we must accept that the same principles apply to mentally handicapped people also. Everyone involved in the care plan, irrespective of discipline or status, is involved in the teaching team. Most importantly, mentally handicapped people themselves have a major role to play in their own education.

1 Conflict

There has always been an element of conflict between teachers and nurses. The differences in the working day of both groups, and the disparity of esteem in conditions and salaries, have helped to foster the conflict further. Having personally worked on both sides of the argument, I can only present the reader with a personal view of the situation. The philosophies of both professional groups vary little. Their respective systems have created and reinforced the differences and divide—not the practitioners. But the practitioners must take responsibility for perpetuating the consequences of that divide. Conflict often arises from misunderstandings and breakdown of communication. In my own experience, I have found that the conflict existing between two professional or non-professional groups stems from a distinct lack of information and knowledge flow between those groups. As long as disciplines train independently from each other, there will be little hope that the systems will come together. *Isolated training produces isolated practitioners.*

The 1982 syllabus states: 'These principles will only be achieved if the nurse has the skills and ability to participate in multidisciplinary teamwork in its fullest skill-sharing sense.' It is not enough that the nurse become familiar with what other disciplines are doing—i.e. that the nurse continually learn from others. 'Fullest skill-sharing sense' stresses the need for nurses to impart their knowledge and share their skills with others involved in the care plan.

Example

The Further Education Unit for 16–19-year-old profoundly handicapped students was situated on the site of a large long-stay hospital. When I first began working there, I was struck by the very obvious lack of communication between the wards and the unit. Apart from 'good morning' and 'good afternoon', there was little else said by nurses and teachers to each other as they escorted students to and from the unit. The day-books that students had conveyed all the factual information, but it was as though nurses and teachers spoke different languages.

Going to the wards early to collect students and spending more time there made little difference in improving relationships between the two staff groups. What we needed to overcome was the threat that we posed to each other. As I saw it, there was only one way to resolve the poor communication. I requested to work an early shift on the ward.

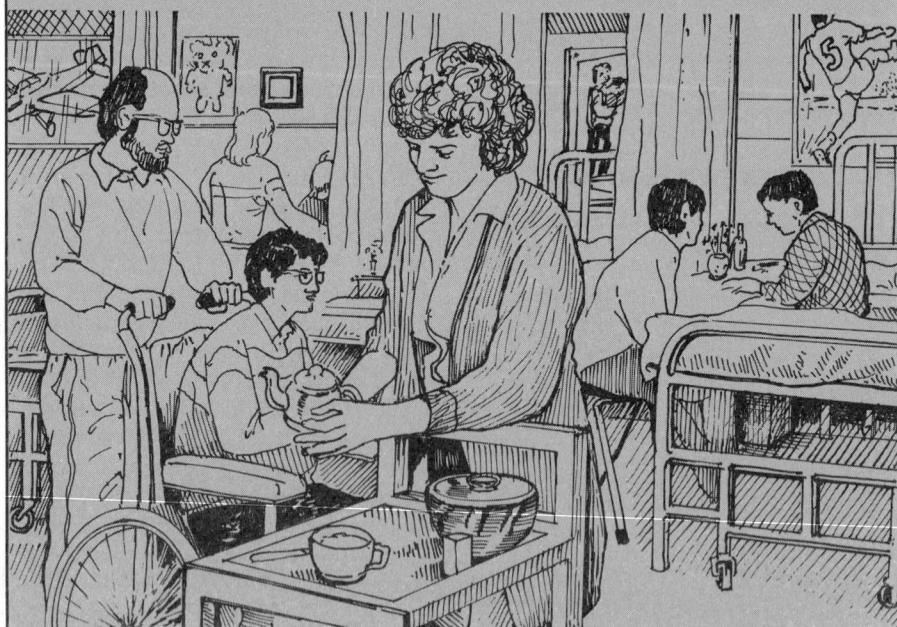

I was most struck by just how much I had forgotten. Not in terms of what to do, but in terms of how it used to feel. I had forgotten how frantic early mornings are; how fraught breakfast time can be; how stressful it is to get everything ready on time.

I was reminded of how unreasonable day-care staff can be when people don't arrive on time. I am not so sure how the nurses felt! But we are all aware now of the need to work together. Those two hours on the ward made all the difference. Feeling that we belonged to the same team, the barriers came down and we began to talk to each other.

Both the teaching team and the nursing team have benefited from the experience already outlined. We have greater understanding, better support and, most importantly, a more cohesive programme for the student whose care we all share.

(c) Teaching what?

Thus far we have briefly discussed the educational process and looked at the importance of learning to trust one another so that we can work together. Now I should like to move on and examine some of the areas and issues that come under the umbrella of teaching. Before we begin this examination of individual programmes, I feel that it is important to establish some focal points.

- The new skill must be 'normal' and in context of daily life.
- The new skill must be in the interests of the individual and not taught to suit the needs of the staff or the system.
- The new skill must not be so specialised that access is withheld from other members of the care team.
- The new skill must be aimed towards independence and not towards creating dependence on the teacher.

These points may appear to be rather obvious, but I feel that they need to be identified, as, unfortunately, they are often overlooked. It is very easy to become lost in the routine and management of an area, and then lose sight of the very things that dictate why we are there.

(d) Respecting individuality

We must never assume that what works for one will work for all. Each person is an individual, with individual needs, and therefore programmes and care plans must reflect this individuality. As much as it is important to recognise the individuality of mentally handicapped people, it is equally important to recognise the individuality of practitioners. Our varied and diverse backgrounds, experiences and outlooks, determine our ways of working and interaction with one another. This, therefore, ultimately affects how we teach. As practitioners we are all under tremendous pressure to be doing something all of the time. We easily become so absorbed in filling the hours of our working days that we end up not doing any teaching at all. If we are tired or frustrated, we will never be able to commit ourselves fully to our teaching. Similarly, if those in our care are having an off-day, they are not going to be responsive to what we have to offer. Timing is all-important. Because we just happen to be there does not mean that learning will automatically take place. Both parties have to be together for learning to be successful and meaningful, and both parties must be honest with each other. Practitioners also have to be able to trust one another. We can pick and choose our friends, but we do not have the same elements of choice at work. Mentally handicapped people are at an even greater disadvantage than we are. Within their respective care settings, they have absolutely no choice in selecting who will care for them.

When we decide to teach something, we must ensure that everyone in the care team has the opportunity to do that teaching. This is not for our benefit. This is to allow mentally handicapped people the opportunity to choose. We, the practitioners, must start with facilitating the widest variables possible, and we must begin with choice.

(e) Environmental teaching

Before we can even start thinking about individual programmes, we must take a long hard look at the environment in which we will do our teaching.

By and large, this has been decided for us. When we look around at our work surroundings, do we give enough thought to the fact that we just have to work there but that, for many, this is their home? We set our own standards for our lives—because we have the choice to do so. We can decide whether we want to sleep in an unmade bed, drink out of chipped cups, eat warm food off cold plates. We can decide whether we want to have a bath every day or every week. Very often, mentally handicapped people in care settings have had these elements of choice taken away from them. Maybe they would like to sit in a different chair, have a new cushion, not have sugar in their tea. Maybe they would like to change the furniture around. Home, supposedly, is where the heart is. Wherever or whatever home may be, then this is where the centre of the educational process ought to take place. We hear an awful lot about 'normalisation' and yet we do the silliest of things in our attempts to introduce it.

Let us now look at what happens at the start of the day and establish just how normal we make it.

When mentally handicapped people wake up in the morning, is it in response to an alarm clock going off on their bedside table? If a survey could be taken to establish just how much time is spent teaching 'time' to mentally handicapped children and adults, I am confident that we would find the results quite staggering and hard to believe. But what is even harder to believe is how we so easily dispense with this subject area. By introducing bedside clocks and watches for individuals, and by having ward and department clocks in accessible places where they can be seen by all (i.e. not near the ceiling), we can extend this 'normal' subject area into the context of daily life. For the profoundly handicapped person, getting dressed in the morning can be an anxious time. The situation is made more stressful because breakfast just will not wait for anyone.

We are all of us familiar with an early morning rush. But even the most hectic of households organises a system to suit the needs of the individuals involved. We can choose to eat breakfast in dressing-gowns, or be ready in time to eat breakfast dressed. We even have the luxury of deciding whether we want to eat breakfast at all. But when we are at work, do we really pay enough attention to the needs of the individual 'household' at breakfast time? The start to the day is very important, because it sets the tone for what follows. It might suit staff to have breakfast over by a certain time—but at what cost? When we are needed to help with dressing, we ought to use this very special one-to-one time to encourage head, arm and leg movements and change of position. In this way the most profoundly handicapped person will feel as if they are contributing to the process and not just leaving it all for the practitioner to do.

When our help is not needed with dressing, we can make good use of this special time to talk about things such as the weather. Temperature influences the way *we* dress and influences *our* choice of clothing. Can we afford to ignore the same influence it has on mentally handicapped people? This is teaching!

Looking after our possessions and our homes is a very basic element of our lives. Having clean linen on our beds and clean clothes to wear, polishing, dusting, hoovering, washing up, emptying waste bins, tidying up—all very normal everyday things. Very normal things that help us to develop a sense of pride in ourselves and our environment. We would not choose to sit on smelly chairs, in lounges devoid in parts of wallpaper, with curtains hanging by just one or two hooks. And because we would not set these standards for ourselves, we cannot sit back and allow them to be that way for people who can't always get up and do something about it. If we get up and involve ourselves in maintaining good standards of household management, this, too, is teaching.

We are able to go round supermarkets and try out all sorts of different foodstuffs and drinks. Just taking tea as an example, there are so many different varieties: lemon, herbal, China, Indian, rosehip, blackcurrant, and so on. We can choose to try them and then decide whether we like them or not. If mentally handicapped people never have the opportunity to try new things,

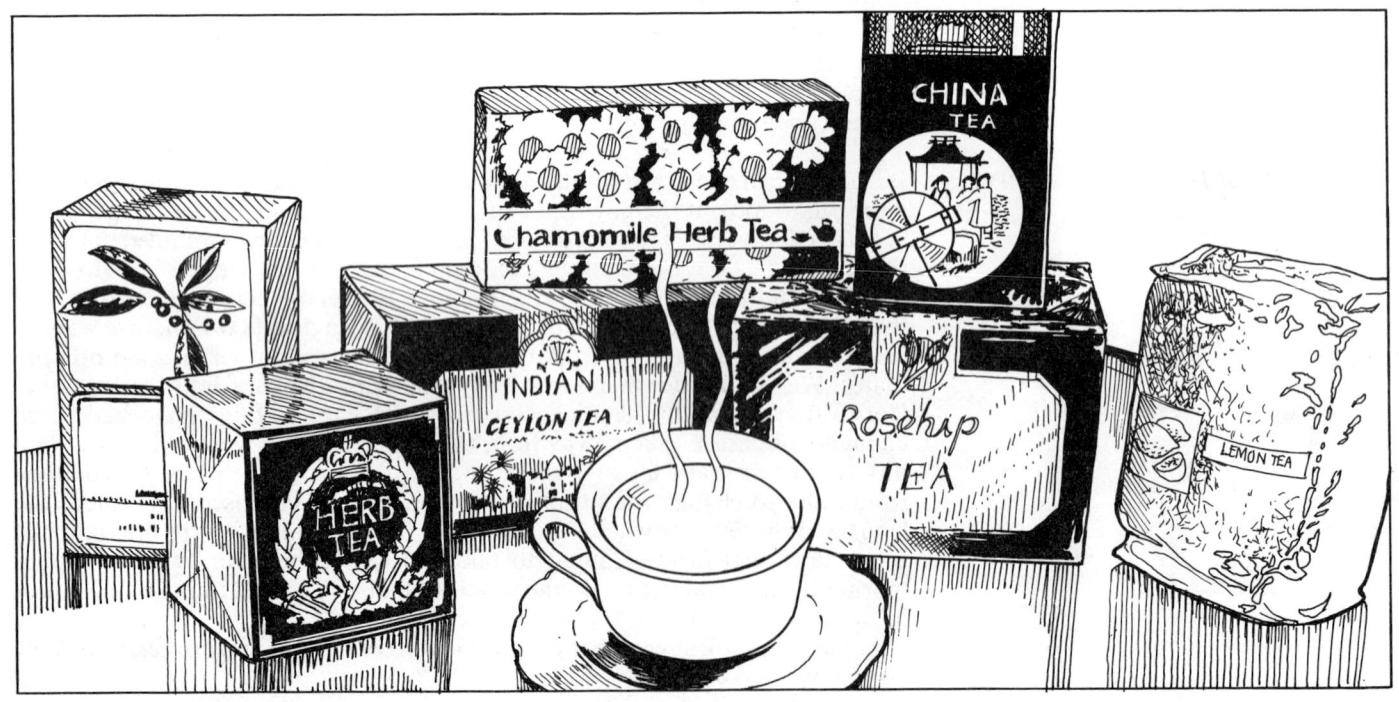

how can they ever have the opportunity to choose? If we are really in the business of widening horizons, things like teatime should not be excluded. Allowing handicapped people the chance to say 'yes' or 'no' is teaching.

At the end of a hard day at work, we choose to spend our leisure time in ways that we prefer. It may well be the same every day—but it may not. We may choose to go to bed early, or we may decide to stay up late. If we could transfer some of this normality to handicapped people in our care, this, too, would be teaching.

(f) Teaching in context

Sometimes *where* we teach hinders *what* we teach. For, as much as there needs to be variety in *what*, so there also needs to be variety in *where* and *when*. As stated earlier, we must be mindful that what we are teaching is normal and in context, and it must have relevance and meaning outside of the teaching setting. We must be careful that we are teaching the right and appropriate things, and not setting double standards.

Example

As part of an overall programme concentrating on independence training, a small group of teenagers were involved in a teeth-cleaning programme each lunch time. The group travelled into town for a hamburger lunch. Having eaten their mid-day meal, they went to the toilet. The entire group had a panic attack when they discovered that individually named toilet bags, containing toothbrushes, paste and face cloths, were not hanging up on individually named pegs.

How much time, effort and energy is wasted on unrealistic teaching?

Guidelines are important. When we start working with mentally handicapped people, we are given a lot of information pertaining to all the things that cannot be done. Given enough time, the newest recruit to the field would be able to draw up a comprehensive list of the 'can't do's'. As educators, what we really need to be concentrating on is the list of 'can do's'.

If we are going to be part of a team which works towards progress, then we must start off with strengths—as well as weaknesses. Very often the weaknesses are obvious—the strengths are not. But if we are unaware of the reality that strengths *are* present, then we are not going to be so receptive to seeing them. It costs very little to make a list at the outset.

Weaknesses

1. Needs help with dressing.
2. Needs help with feeding.
3. Incontinent.
4. Screams often.
5. Will bang objects against head.
6. Refuses to do anything when asked.
7. Dislikes noise.
8. Becomes agitated when routine is upset.

Strengths

1. Some control over head and arms.
2. When spoon is loaded, can co-ordinate it to mouth unaided.
3. Favourite drink is coffee.
4. Relaxes completely when being massaged.
5. Smiles spontaneously when playing with water.
6. Enjoys having time to himself.
7. Makes good eye contact when being read a story.
8. Can recognise some members of staff and peer group.
9. Anticipates some activities well.
10. Given a favourite series of pictures can visually scan well.
11. Good head movement and neck control when having hair dried.

This list could be almost endless. What we need to concentrate on is our ability to use the strengths to overcome the weaknesses.

Case notes are full of information. It is important to be familiar with previous history and previous reports—but it must not stop there. We all view people in different ways, and things do change from day to day. So it is very important to have an up-to-date and clear picture of what is going on. The information gathered, plus the new information from each day, must be accessible and available for all members of the care team. Inevitably this puts 'communication' to the test. We must not presume that because *we* know what's there, everyone else will automatically be as well informed.

In drawing up care plans, we need to include all the very normal things of everyday life as part of those plans. As we have outlined strengths and weaknesses of those we are caring for, so we must draw up lists of *our* strengths and weaknesses. We cannot presume that we are all going to be able to teach everything—and teach it well. We, too, will have subject areas that we feel comfortable with and areas that we know little about. All this needs to be discussed openly—not so that the *best* do the teaching, but the most *appropriate*.

Those of us who lack the experience or opportunity must ask to be educated by those who do know. This will spread skills, provide variety and halt stagnation. We cannot afford to cocoon ourselves away into the safety of our respective disciplines. Although training courses are at last becoming more comprehensive, we are still a long way off having one discipline that knows it all. If we don't start to cross over one another's boundaries, and find out more, then we are deliberately withholding expertise and experience from the very people who need to benefit from it.

Example

Julie had recently returned to her long-stay ward in a large institution, following extensive orthopaedic investigation and treatment. At the very top of the priority list was an intensive physiotherapy programme which had to be completed every day. At the time, Julie was 18 years old and attending an Education Unit five days each week. The day-to-day demands of the ward staff, coupled with low staffing levels, made it impossible for Julie's programme to be completed each morning in time for her to attend the unit. This resulted in her not attending at all. To facilitate the new programme, within the existing framework, necessitated a number of disciplines working something out between them. Nursing and teaching staff familiarised themselves with the programme—both groups being supervised by the physiotherapists.

Instead of the exercises replacing the educational programme, they

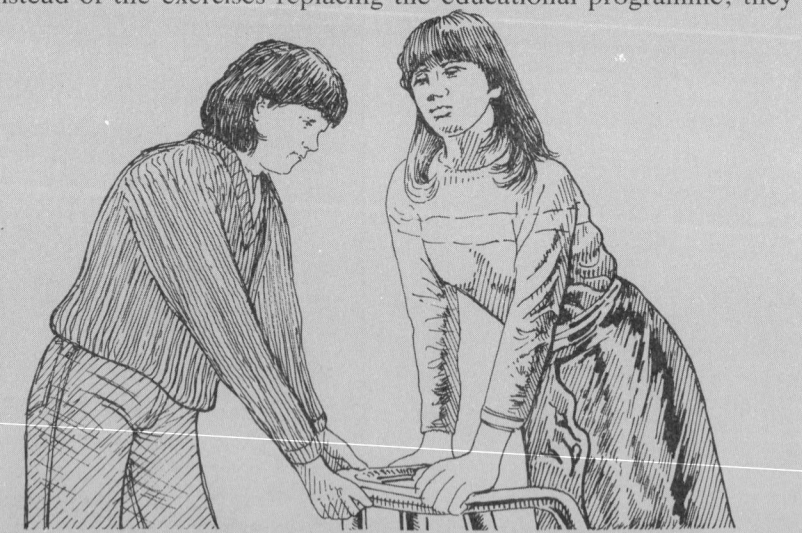

became the focal point. Pressure was taken off ward staff Monday to Friday. The nursing staff carried out the programme over weekends, when routines were not as fraught. Julie responded well to the consistency of her exercises and her mobility improved greatly. When in her Flexi stand, we were able to continue Julie's one-to-one work. The only difference was that now we had to do it all standing up! How could we not have shared one another's roles? When we did share, we found tremendous support from one another. No one party felt overloaded or put upon. We were able to put Julie's needs before our own, irrespective of 'role'.

(g) Now we're teaching . . . now what?

Having looked at the areas we need to be concentrating on, and the resources of the staff team, we can then put the programme into action. Implementation of programmes is a subject area that has been dealt with by other authors and is beyond the remit of this chapter. However, I should like to remind the reader of two key points:

- Teaching must be 'normal'.
- Teaching must be in context.

If we can carry these two points into our working day, we will have an excellent base for effective teaching programmes.

If the educational process is to be ongoing and progressive, then practitioners must be ongoing and progressive too. It simply will not do to implement a programme and then run that programme for ever. There may be aspects of that programme which need to continue, but we need to be mindful about preventing programmes from becoming boring and repetitive. Just as it is important to monitor the progress of mentally handicapped people, so it is equally important to monitor and evaluate the programme in operation. To evaluate successfully what we have been doing, we need to be honest. We need to be able to admit to our failings—as well as our successes. It does not necessarily follow that if progress is not being made, the fault lies with the mentally handicapped person. It is far more probable that the fault lies with the programme and the practitioner. Regular discussions must take place to keep abreast of new information and to facilitate the opportunity for sharing ideas and thoughts. Above all, the programme must be realistic and centred entirely around the needs of the individual concerned.

Example

James, a young man of 22 years, lived at home with his parents. To correct and maintain his scoliosis, it was necessary for him to wear a body brace. This was very tight-fitting and, not surprisingly, created constant pressure on his abdomen when worn. Jame's incontinence problems followed no set pattern. Some days he would stay dry all morning—other days he needed changing three or four times.

James had had a very rigid toilet training programme from a very early age, which had continued throughout his time in Special School. This had

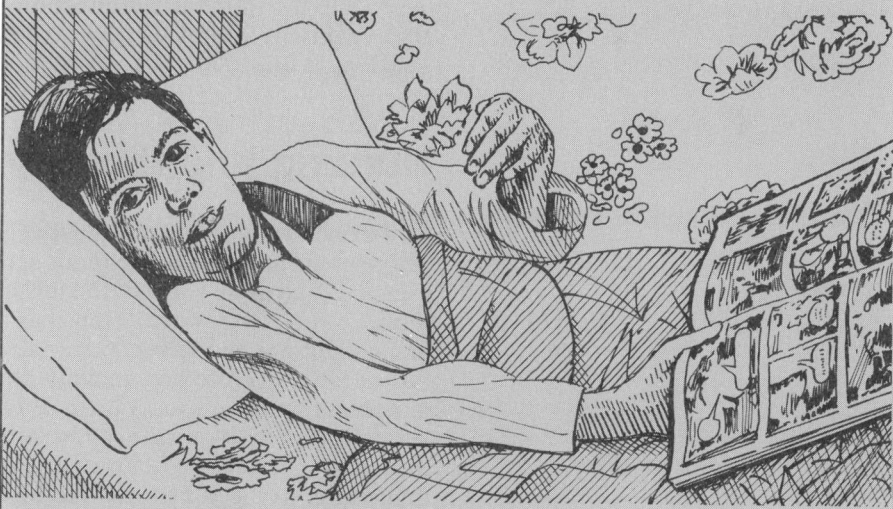

taken up an enormous amount of time and effort by both James and teaching staff.

James's incontinence was not because he was *unteachable*—but because he wore a brace. To have continued with James's toilet programme would only have created more anxieties. The most important factor was that James did not suffer from any undue discomfort—i.e. stay wet for long periods of time. Rather than pursue 'the toilet programme', we tried to build-in a more normal pattern of teaching. On arrival at the Unit, James's brace was 'checked', and he was given the choice of going to the toilet. This allowed James ten minutes to be free of the brace—something seen by James as being a treat. Because we appeared to be

Continued

> concentrating on the brace, this allowed a much lower profile to be taken with regard to the incontinence problem.
>
> We were aware of how much time James would have to spend during the day being 'handled' in terms of taking the brace off and putting it back on, if we were to continue with a two-hourly toilet programme. It seemed to make more sense to limit this to three times during the day.
>
> When James was incontinent, we could not blame him for being lazy or not signing that he wanted to go to the toilet. The practitioners had prescribed something that added to the incontinence problem and so the practitioners had to find a way of dealing with it. It would have been most unfair to have subjected this young man to a training programme which compensated for staff decisions.

(h) Extending our role

The role of the nurse as educator is not confined to teaching mentally handicapped people. The nurse, alongside other disciplines involved, has a responsibility to educate much wider circles.

There are a great many people in daily contact with mentally handicapped people who have absolutely no idea what's going on. There are ever-increasing numbers of administrators making very important decisions about standards of care and types of provision, but without any real understanding of the implications their decision-making has—for carers or for the cared for.

While we are working hard to protect the dignity and self-respect of handicapped people, we are still surrounded by great numbers of people involved who, unfortunately, do not share those same beliefs.

We must find ways to extend our role as educator, so that we can reach those great numbers whose attitudes, behaviour and short-sightedness hinders the work we are doing.

People who make mocking remarks and hurtful comments about handicapped people only persist in doing so because no one has told them to stop. No one has told them that it's not OK to keep saying those things. Sometimes we forget that colleagues and peers in our own home base have lost touch with what's going on. Yes, we need to prepare and educate the community, but we still have a lot of work to do at home.

The role of the nurse as educator has to have the degree of flexibility needed to be able to stretch in all directions and across all boundaries. The skills to achieve this are within very easy reach. Teaching is not mysterious or complex. Teaching is quite simply good common-sense.

Nursing and therapy

At the outset it must be stressed that all that this heading entails cannot possibly be discussed fully within the remit of this chapter. But what I should like to do is principally clear up some of the misunderstandings surrounding therapy. Over recent years, the word itself has developed certain mystical qualities—misconceptions and misunderstandings have therefore been almost inevitable. As therapy, even today, remains, by and large, grossly misrepresented and misinterpreted, so, too, is the role of the therapist.

Both inside and outside of the nursing profession, the confusion over 'what therapy is' prevails. So before we can even begin to explore how therapy relates to nursing, we need first of all to be absolutely sure of what therapy means.

'Therapy' is not a new word recently introduced into our vocabulary. Derived from the Greek word, *therapeuō*, meaning 'to heal', 'to take care of', 'to tend', it has been in use for centuries. We can therefore safely say that therapy is the treatment or cure for disorder.

Each culture interprets disorder in different ways. The Swiss regarded the birth of a handicapped baby born into a family as being a good sign—a favour from Heaven. The Ancient Greeks believed that epilepsy was a sign that there was communication with the gods. Presumably, for both of these examples, there was no need for therapy. How times change.

If therapy is the treatment or cure for disorder, then the therapist must be the person who cares/heals/treats/takes care of this disorder. Isn't this what all nurses are trained to do? So why is the nurse not seen as being the therapist to the sick person?

The general public regard nurses as being those people in the caring profession who see to the everyday needs of the sick person. That is to say, the 'sick' person in a 'sick' place. The traditional role is that of the patient in bed, with the nurse in attendance. Other disciplines may come and go but the nurse is always there.

The changing role of the nurse has been evident for a great number of years. Evident, that is, to nurses—not so to the general public. Psychiatric nurses *nurse* very few of their patients in bed. Very few of their patients actually *look* ill. But nurses working in the field of mental handicap have no very clear outward role for the general public. A great many people still believe that nursing mentally handicapped people means either minding and supervising, or caring (in the sick sense) for the most profoundly handicapped sector of the community. All nurses, irrespective of chosen field, undertake the physical care of those in their charge. When patients recover, or when the disorder or sickness is brought under control, nurses are seen as being the key people responsible for bringing about these changes. But the change is primarily seen as being a *physical and outward* change.

To know and understand where we are at now, we need to know and understand where we have come from. As we look back through the ages and decades at the historical background of respective disciplines and professions, we can compare areas of common ground and areas of shared concern. The caring professions have one major area of common concern—that of caring. But the ways in which the different disciplines have set about their respective caring are as diverse as the number of disciplines and professions involved. A great deal overlaps—but a great deal still remains stereotyped and categorised.

It is within this whole aspect of 'caring' that confusion over therapy arises. We are all of us capable listeners—an important skill for all nurses to have. But being good listeners does not make us therapists. We can provide a shoulder to cry on—but that does not make us therapists either. We can advise, support and encourage—again, this does not make us therapists. We may find ourselves counselling handicapped people, their relatives, their peers, our colleagues—a frequent occurrence maybe, but not a therapeutic one.

Setting aside our professional hats for a while, and moving outside of the work environment, let us now take a brief look at some of the roles familiar to us, which could easily be seen as being 'therapeutic', but clearly are not.

- Someone close to us loses a member of his family and is clearly disturbed by the bereavement. He comes to us for consolation and solace. We allow time and space for his grief to have some outlet—and we listen as long as we have to, the listening being the way in which we can offer the most appropriate help.
- We have a bad day at work. Getting off to the wrong start, we have gone from one crisis to another; the pressure has been unrelenting. On arrival home, we offload—to someone, anyone, who happens to be there: or the dog, the cat, the budgie. Working households start their end of working day by sharing the pleasure and pain of the day.
- An elderly relative is ill and is going into hospital for routine tests. Unsure about what is wrong, he is convinced that whatever is wrong is terminal, and that he will never leave the ward alive. We give reassurance, send cards and flowers, and offer lots of support.
- A neighbour has been incapacitated and unable to go shopping. We pop round and offer to do their shopping, post letters and see to any other jobs which may need doing.
- A friend with two small children has been invited to an evening function and cannot go because of baby-sitter problems. We offer to sit to enable her to go.
- A couple we have known for years split up. Both parties are extremely upset. We offer our support to both: phone calls, invites for a meal, and long conversations into the small hours.

The list of examples could be never-ending. In all these cases we don't stop and think about what it is we are doing—we just do it. It is all part of the very normal and natural way in which we care for those around us. We often feel that, were the tables turned, we would only hope that someone would be there for us should we need her. We must not confuse this natural and inner sense of caring we have with any therapeutic model.

My personal feelings are that it is within this very area that the confusion lies—not just from the nurse's standpoint, but from that of other disciplines as well. There is predominantly the misleading notion that 'to do what therapists do' is therapy.

(a) So what do therapists do?

Before they do anything, they are trained. Although training varies, people entering therapy training, as a general rule, do so with the added perspective of a previously acquired related professional background and training. In other words, school-leavers cannot leave school to become therapists.

During training, the therapist will be taught the theoretical base, and be exposed to the experiential aspects of working therapeutically. Training involves an undertaking of personal therapy. The combination of these three elements makes training lengthy, demanding and arduous. Although assessment is ongoing, in most cases supervised practice and a great deal of written work and examinations are necessary to qualify. If there are any doubts as to the suitability of practitioners in training, qualification and licence to practice is withheld. Having trained and qualified, the therapist then goes into practice. But it does not stop there. The processes learned become an ongoing methodology for daily use—and the therapist will use the resources of the therapeutic network to retain clear vision and sense of direction. Often this will involve regular supervised sessions and attendance at workshops. Unlike many other disciplines, the hard work in therapy starts when the training stops.

Therapists will put forward the argument that they are the facilitators for bringing about internal change. They have been trained to acknowledge and experience their own internal change, and therefore have insight, understanding and empathy with the internal changes of others.

Nurses can argue that they, too, are facilitators of internal change—and they are, by the very nature of their level and depth of caring. The relationships and bonding which develop between nurses and those in their care, especially in the field of handicap, can be extremely close. At times it is impossible to be 'distant'. I am not ashamed to admit to 'loving' the young people I work with. The 'love' comes from the friendship which has grown with time. As with all relationships, 'love' can be a hidden but important element. Being 'loved' makes a difference to our lives.

For handicapped people, being 'loved' can give a meaning to life. If they can feel 'loved' and supported, this in itself can bring about internal changes. But it should be stressed that this natural change is something quite separate from therapeutic change. To list the different *types* of therapy would warrant another book. My personal view is that there is a time and a place for everything, and I believe that therapists do have an important part to play in the care of handicapped people.

If 'therapy' or 'care' or 'treatment' has been prescribed as an appropriate measure for the particular needs of a person at that given time, then so long as it *is* appropriate, that's fine. But what very often happens is that when the people who make the decisions have exhausted the more traditional forms of 'treatment', that's the time they call in the therapist.

(b) The nurse working with the therapist

No one discipline has all the answers. There may be those who think they do, but the reality is that they don't. All the disciplines involved in the care of handicapped people are needed, but there are no hard and fast rules which dictate that one is more important or relevant than another.

The nurse, at the outset, must realise that all the skills needed to provide a holistic approach to care will not be made available to them throughout their training. The syllabus is very comprehensive, but is by no means complete. It is equally important to remember that other disciplines, too, including therapists, have bits missing from their training programmes. To have formalised training which would include everything that practitioners need would result in ten-year training programmes, at least!

Although we must envisage that in years to come training will undergo radical change, we are still left with what we do today. The nurse, whether in training or qualified, has a responsibility to those in her care to ensure that everything possible is being done to improve quality of life.

The nurse and the therapist need each other. Many of their skills are interlinked and need to be shared. For the handicapped person, they need to see that practitioners are all on the same side—*their* side: that they are not two people who work in isolation. If we could put ourselves in the shoes of that handicapped person, how would we feel if two people kept telling us that they are there to make us feel better—and yet they can't even talk to each other or know what each other is doing? If the therapist is working in a predominantly 'nursing' area, then it makes sense for the nurse to know what's going on, and that is not going to be achieved through isolation. Therapists don't bite!

(c) Becoming professional

Nurse education affords the student time and opportunity to do all sorts of things that can't be fitted in once qualified! Although many new experiences may not make much sense at the time, the nursing student must take advantage of all the situations which come her way to enable her to gain insight into new areas of work. As her work progresses, and new pieces of the jigsaw are slotted into place, an overall widening of horizons will develop quite naturally.

Students can also ask lots of questions. In my experience, it seems as if once qualified = knows it all! I find it very surprising that qualified staff feel uneasy about asking questions. If the subject area is unfamiliar, then why on earth ought they to know the answers anyway?

Being professional is being able to admit to not knowing. This is not an admission of failure on the part of the practitioner: it shows that the practitioner cares enough to find out more.

The therapist has a great deal to offer—to both clients and staff. Nurses would be well advised to regard therapists as allies and not as the enemy. How nurses go about this is, of course, a matter for each individual to decide.

The only way to know what therapy is about is to experience it! There are, of course, libraries full of books on the subject, and it is important to read the literature—but you can't beat the real thing. Readers interested in pursuing this further should try to participate in some therapy workshops. There are now a great many workshops set up specifically for practitioners working in the field of handicap, and these are proving to be in great demand. Apart from the practical experience gained, they are extremely useful in terms of bringing people together—to share ideas and problems and reduce the risk of professional isolation.

Courses and workshops are usually advertised in relevant periodicals and magazines. For readers working in the same environment as therapists, why not make a start on the building of bridges by asking them to put you on their mailing lists? You might also write to the major organisations and ask to be kept informed of latest news/conferences/workshops, etc.

Launching into therapy training is something that needs to be given very careful consideration. It is also important to ensure that you are fully aware of what it entails. By participating in a variety of workshops, you will be better equipped to make the right decision. Looking up 'therapy' in the library index ought to at least throw some light on the complexity and enormity of the subject area.

But whatever you decide to do, or not do, the most important point is that the service we offer to mentally handicapped people must meet their needs. Whether we are nurses, teachers or therapists, those needs ought to determine and dictate how we care.

As mentioned earlier, we cannot afford the luxury of believing that any one discipline has all the answers and all the skills to bring this about. *Nursing* mentally handicapped people is not enough—we have to go much further than that.

Further reading

Borger, R. and Seaborne, A. E. M., *The Psychology of Learning*, 2nd edn, Penguin, 1982

Brudenell, P., *The Other Side of Profound Handicap*, Macmillan Education, 1986

Burr, L. A. (ed.), *Therapy Through Movement*, Nottingham Rehab Ltd, 1986

Cottam, P. J. and Sutton, A. (eds), *Conductive Education*, Croom Helm, 1986

Holt, J., *How Children Fail*, Penguin, 1968

Holt, J., *How Children Learn*, Penguin, 1970

Jennings, S., *Remedial Drama*, Pitman, 1973; reprinted Black, 1981

Jennings, S. (ed.), *Creative Therapy*, Pitman 1975; reprinted Kemble Press, 1983

Jennings, S., *Creative Drama In Group Work*, Winslow Press, 1986

Jennings, S. (ed.), *Dramatherapy Theory and Practice: A Source Book for Clinicians and Teachers*, Croom Helm, 1987

Levete, G., *No Handicap to Dance*, Souvenir Press, 1982

McClintock, A., *Drama for Mentally Handicapped Children*, Souvenir Press, 1984

Pavey, D., *Art Based Games*, Methuen, 1979

Chapter 8

Research-mindedness in client care

by Tom Keighley

In the Foreword to *Research for Nursing* (MacLeod Clarke and Hockey, 1979), Majorie Simpson wrote:

> 'The 1980s hold at least three major challenges. The first must be met by researchers moving to more difficult areas of work and extracting from the theories and methods of the sciences allied to nursing those aspects which are meaningful in a nursing setting and, as necessary, developing unique approaches to the study of nursing care. The second is the responsibility of the whole profession to use the findings of research, balancing them with professional judgement for the advancement of the practice of nursing. The third is to marry the two in a true partnership between research and practice.'

Research-mindedness is best defined as the last two of Miss Simpson's challenges. The fact that the nursing profession is entering the latter half of the decade she described does not detract from the urgency of addressing those challenges.

Understanding research is an activity that few of the half million or so practising nurses in the UK will ever master. It is a specialist activity with its own knowledge base, skills and attitudes. It is only an elite activity in as much as any other nursing specialism is, be it behaviour therapy or stoma care. However, it is a specialist activity, and not something to be dabbled in without appropriate training and supervision. In contrast, all nurses should as part of their basic nursing education acquire the skills to be research-minded. The question, then, is twofold:

1. How to become research-minded?
2. How to nurse in a research-minded manner?

How to become research-minded

In order to become research-minded, a number of well-established skills have to be acquired and practised regularly. It is rather like typing: by failing to practise at frequent intervals, one soon forgets where the letters are. These abilities are not in any hierarchical order, but include the following:

- Learning to access research.
- Acquiring a basic numeracy.
- Developing an advanced level of critical reasoning.
- Understanding the use of different research methods.
- Evaluating the ethics of research projects.
- The ability to evaluate the usefulness of a piece of research.
- The conceptual skills which enable a research problem to be identified.

While this may appear a formidable list, the basic elements of each of these skills are present in all those who enter nurse education. The art is to develop the skills to such a level that they become part of the unconscious mechanisms at work in the mind of the caring nurse. However, there are separate elements to each skill, and while they come to overlap in practice, they can certainly be learnt and practised separately to begin with.

(a) Accessing research

Research is: 'An attempt to increase available knowledge by the discovery of new facts through scientific enquiry' (Macleod Clarke and Hockey, 1979). It is the hallmark of an organised mind that an individual spends some time, even if it is only a moment, clarifying the objectives of an exercise. It is very important, therefore, to know clearly what it is that access is being sought to. While some would argue with the appropriateness of the definition, especially if they use 'softer' research methods such as ethnographic techniques which centre on observation of populations, this definition has much merit. First, it acknowledges that research is intended to increase the knowledge base on any particular subject. Second, as a process, research is an attempt to generate new facts, the so-called building blocks of knowledge. Third, these facts are generated through scientific enquiry—i.e. the application of objective and systematic processes which others can learn and, where necessary, repeat.

Importantly, the definition does not denigrate or undermine the significance of the other source of knowledge. This is the subjective knowledge which is based on experience, and consisting of the rational review of events and the application of internal logical processes to one's conscious world. However, research often has a role to play here, as subjective assumptions can often be tested objectively. The findings of such research permit the individual to place in a wider context his or her previous beliefs and understanding. With this definition, one should also realise that nursing research is no different from any other form of research. Systematic scientific enquiry is practised in many disciplines, and this has great implications for nurses working in mental handicap.

Too often, students of nursing come to believe that their concern should be only with research done *by* nurses. This is simply not so. There is much to be gained from work completed in all the social sciences, in psychology and education, in straight physics and chemistry, and in physiology and medicine. This does not discount the work undertaken by nurse researchers, but it does reveal the size of the task when accessing research. It means that nursing libraries, which should be the primary source for any literature review process, should not only contain standard textbooks, but should also be concentrating their resources on the most relevant journals to the discipline they are serving. This should be facilitated by the appointment of a qualified librarian. No one else is prepared to anything like the same degree to help the student obtain the information she wants or to acquaint the student with what information is available.

1 Learning to use the library

In accessing research, therefore, the two primary skills to acquire are identifying good libraries and learning how to use them. Learning how to use a library is time-consuming but not something to be dismissed lightly. The library is a treasure-house of knowledge and information. A nurse without library skills is like a blind person without a guide-dog, open to the greatest dangers so easily avoided by those with vision. These skills include:

- Knowing the book and journal categorisation.
- Being able to trace material through the index system either on computer, microfiche or cards.
- Understanding how the libraries can assist when difficulties arise.

It will not be long before work on an index suggests that a second level of skills is required. This relates to the words used to describe things. For example, 'care of the incontinent patient' to one author is 'the maintenance of continence' to another; 'care of the individual with a mental handicap' in the UK usually reads in the United States as 'care of mental defectives'. While the terms 'imbecile' and 'idiot' are now terms of abuse in Britain, in some parts of the English-speaking world they are still formal diagnostic terms. The point being made here is that before starting to search, a thesaurus-type exercise is required. All possible terms should be identified and meanings reviewed as the search continues. Most confusion is caused by lack of precision in meaning. Learning to be clear in thought and expressions is a large part of being research-minded.

The next phase is what to do with the information found. This is where 6 in × 8 in cards come into their own—computers are even better, if available. The card (even if on computer) should contain the following information:
- The title of the work, starting with the keyword—e.g. 'Nursing the Incontinent Patient' becomes 'Incontinent Patient, Nursing the'.
- Author's name and date—e.g. Grace, W. A. (1982).

- Source of information—e.g. *Nursing Times*, **73** (Oct. 27), pp. 34–42.
- Content, including nature of study, size of sample, findings, limitations identified by author.
- Your own comments on the source.

This is then filed in your own index.

The student having read as widely as possible, should produce a summary paper, even if no one has requested it. This completes the discipline of attempting to discover knowledge. It prepares the student for a further stage in her research-mindedness development—i.e critical thinking, which is addressed a little further on in the text.

In order to facilitate the earlier process of gaining access to research, some nurses have found it possible to create an access file. From their weekly reading of journals, articles and books, they note on individual 6 in × 4 in or even 5 in × 3 in cards interesting sources. Two cards are made out, one listing the subject, by the keyword technique, and another card listing the author(s). This takes a few minutes each week, but converts the gentle browse through a journal into a constructive activity which helps to build into the mind a cognate map of the nursing knowledge the individual has tapped into.

(b) Acquiring a basic numeracy

Few nurses in any discipline of nursing are ever heard to boast about their facility with numbers. Researchers are no different from other nurses in this respect. They, too, often struggle with the mathematics in their studies. In order to help them, they nearly always involve a statistician in their work. Indeed, in larger studies, so important is the statistician that it is difficult to know at what point in the research process the statistician's skills can be ignored.

However, in emphasising the importance of the statistician, it is not right to conclude that nurses have no need to question the numbers in a study where a statistician has been involved. Neither is it correct to conclude that only a specialist can acquire the skills required to review the numerical part of a study. Rather, the establishment of a degree of uncertainty about basic numeracy among many nurses has led to a mystique being created about anything to do with numbers. It is important, therefore, to demystify numbers in general, and statistics in particular.

Few nurses have as great a problem with numbers as they suggest. Most can do the basic arithmetic required to check whether they have been overcharged when doing their regular grocery shopping. Similarly, they can perform the additions and subtractions required to calculate whether their monthly salary is correct on their pay slip. Further, they have the ability when out shopping to perform the enormously complicated division and multiplication required to calculate which package of washing powder to buy when the difference in package weight is a few grams and in cost a few pence. The techniques demonstrated in these arithmetical manoeuvres are the sum total of the knowledge required to review the statistics in a research study. Four techniques are required. The reader must be able to:

- Add.
- Subtract.
- Multiply.
- Divide.

That is the sum of the mystery of statistics!

Irvine *et al.* (1979), in the introduction to their book *Demystifying Social Statistics*, note that some people are inherently suspect of statistics because there is: 'a tradition reinforced in popular lore by the tendency to discuss statistics as merely a way of putting one over on people by bewildering them with complicated numbers and mathematics'. They emphasise throughout their text that with a very basic understanding of numbers it is quite possible to perform a quite adequate review; but, also, that the presence of numbers should not reduce the reader either to complete cynicism or complete faith in the study being considered. Rather, the presence of any numerical calculation should result in renewed determination to read closely what is being presented. Experience suggests that a table of numbers compared with an equal amount of text will require three to four times as much time to read, check and finally understand. It is a process which requires great patience and much practice until a degree of facility is acquired. Numeracy for the review of research is not complex, but it requires that the reader be prepared to put into effect the skills acquired by hard practice.

(c) Developing critical reasoning

Critical reasoning is much more than asking questions, though that is part of it. It is more to do with what might be described as the 'If . . . therefore' syndrome. It is the ability to deduce that *if* certain factors pertain, it is right to conclude that *therefore* certain outcomes can be expected, or relationships between things predicted. When reading research, this 'if . . . therefore' approach is absolutely vital. Too often, nurses believe what is presented to them because it is in a book or because it has been written by a famous person. Critical reasoning moves the reader away from all these distractions and irrelevant factors. It forces the reviewer to make judgements purely on the basis of what is in front of him, and to evaluate his findings completely on the logic of the text he is reading.

This will take him through a number of phases. Initially, there is the need to see whether the study makes sense and is feasible as described. There have been a number of instances where research reports have been found to be, at least in part, complete fabrication. At least two Nobel prize winners have been found to have fabricated their results. Questions about their results arose because the claims in the studies did not seem feasible and therefore the studies were repeated. On replication the claims were found to be false. The trigger, however, arose from critical reasoning which suggested that the results were not feasible.

The next stage is to review the objectivity of the researcher. This is one attempt to discover the biases and prejudices that the researcher may not have accounted for in writing up the report of the studies. It should also identify the compromises made in the study, as problems of resource, availability, access to subjects, control of the environment and the external influence of the research supervisor(s) all come to affect the way in which the researcher undertook the study. As the perfect study has yet to be designed and undertaken, the researcher should report these influences or identify why they did not arise.

Applying this critical reasoning approach to evaluating research reports will reveal much to the attentive reader. However, the discovery of illogicalities in a study does not automatically condemn it out of hand. It may still be useful as a guide for particular elements arising out of the study or as points that subsequent researchers should avoid.

(d) Understanding the use of different research methods

For too long, research has been undertaken in a vacuum. Little attempt has been made to base studies within a particular theory or to speculate at the end of the study how the findings influence theory development. The importance of the theory is that it sets a framework which permits the relationship between facts to be established. Failure to demonstrate that relationship will often be the criterion for rejecting a hypothesis or for attempting some new theory-building which accounts for the relationship. This then leads into a further round of testing to check the nature of those relationships. Treece and Treece (1982) demonstrate the relationship like this:

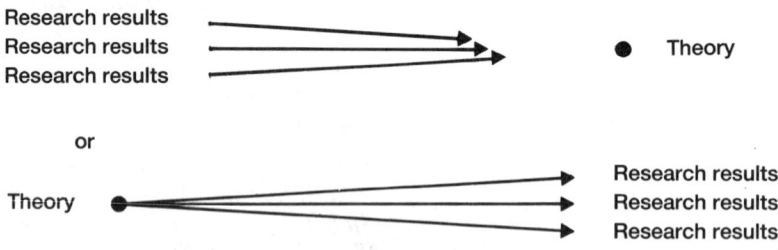

It is important to realise that there is no correct or preferred way, simply an alternative way. In reviewing research, it is important, therefore, to establish where the study fits into this process, and the question needs to be asked—is it based on a theory or is it theory-generating? Arising out of this consideration of theory, it is appropriate to review the research approach adopted. Different reviewers will classify the approach in different ways. However, a quite straightforward line is to categorise the approach under one of five headings: survey, experiment, case study, ethnography or historical. Each approach has different strengths and weaknesses and is more or less appropriate, given the problem being researched. Further, each approach can adopt many different forms, depending on the objective of the study. In nursing, it has not been possible to decide which is or is not the most appropriate approach. The pursuit of a nursing research methodology has for some become a search for the Holy Grail. Increasingly, it is apparent that it is more important to make the approach fit the problem than to constrain the problem to fit the approach.

This line of attack does not in any way limit the range of techniques open to the researcher. The nature of the study problem may require that different methods be adopted, all within one approach, or that findings be triangulated (i.e. checked against one another by the use of different techniques). As with the different approaches, so there are five basic techniques, all of which can be modified: the study of records, observation of subjects, questionnaires, interviewing and experiments.

The question that a reviewer must ask therefore is: 'Which method(s) is (are) most suitable for each research approach?' (Treece and Treece, 1982). The reviewer must, of course, have developed a basic knowledge of the approaches and the techniques. It is the application of the correct approach and technique which resolves problems in research terms. The judgement made is based not only on the knowledge of those approaches and techniques, but also on knowledge of the problem and the subjects under investigation.

(e) The ethics of research

To many nurses, the subject of ethics is as confusing as research can be. At one level, the question of what ethics is can easily be answered by seeing it as the study of those aspects of human behaviour which relate to the rightness or wrongness of that behaviour. However, despite the existence of codes of behaviour (e.g. the laws of the land or the Ten Commandments), what is considered acceptable in human behaviour often changes over time or from place to place. To add to the confusion, an individual may be exposed to contradictory or conflicting guides, or it may even be that the ethical code of a group he or she respects permits a form of behaviour that his or her own professional group rejects. These conflicts are the subject of study by moral philosophers, something which often leaves everyone else feeling that it is inappropriate to pass comment, or maybe judgement.

This position overlooks two important factors. First, that as part of growing up adults have acquired a moral code, no matter how conscious or sub-conscious it is, which directs their behaviour and their judgements on behaviour. Second, that, as nurses, we are guided in our actions by a code of conduct. The existence of these two factors indicates that, as nurses, it is imperative that a review of our own professional ethics be undertaken, not least in the field of nursing research. The Royal College of Nursing Research Society published a document entitled *Ethics Related to Research in Nursing* in 1977. This (at the time of writing) is under review in an attempt to offer guidance based on clear ethical principles rather than simply a list of do's and don'ts. The work of Ian Thompson and others in the United Kingdom suggests that three principles need to be considered:

1. Dignity (right of the individual).
2. Beneficence (well being).
3. Justice.

The problem in the past seems to have been that while one of these three principles might have been considered, they have not always been used in combination.

For example, while some researchers may have considered the autonomy of the research subject, problems of privacy and confidentiality, and the obtaining of consent, were rarely reviewed as a principle. Maybe it was part of nursing's task orientation, but the various aspects of diginity were rarely considered together.

An even more profound difficulty arises around the notion of beneficence (well-being). Research codes in the disciplines of psychology and the social sciences indicate that the value of the findings should outweigh the possible harm that may befall the subject, as one acceptable criterion for doing research. Implicit in this argument is the fact that knowledge for its own sake can be more important than research subjects. This has given rise to a weaker ethical principle—non-malfeasance, made famous by Hippocrates with the dictum, 'First, do no harm'. The challenge for nurses, however, is much greater than that posed by 'doing no harm'. Not only can the nurse be held accountable for failing to prevent harm (non-malfeasance) befalling the patient or client in her care (see UKCC Code, 1984), but also, in the preamble to the code, it is made clear that it is the well-being (beneficence) of the patient or client that is central to nursing practice:

'Each registered nurse, midwife and health visitor shall act at all times in such a manner as to justify public trust and confidence, to uphold and enhance the good standing and reputation of the profession, to serve the interest of society, *and above all to safeguard the interest of individual patients and clients.'* [my italics]

This makes very clear to all nurses that, first and foremost, a nurse is always to be guided by concerns for the well-being of the patient, even, in this case, if the nurse is acting as a researcher. The code makes it clear that the nurse's responsibility extends to the activities of others in relation to the patient (Section 10). Consequently, all nurses must know enough about research to judge whether the project will harm the patient in any way at all.

This brings into play the third principle, i.e. justice, or fairness. It has long been held that it is unfair to do research on certain groups on society. This includes children, the elderly, those with a mental handicap and those with a mental illness. The reason for this is that individuals in these groups are believed to be either less able to give their consent to involvement in research or more susceptible to the pressures researchers may bring to bear on them. The principle of justice leads one to review this actively. For the purposes of the research proposed, it might be appropriate not to involve individuals from these groups, but the question raised by the principle of justice is whether fairness to one person or one group does or does not lead to unfairness to other persons or groups. For example, if it is considered appropriate to undertake research into genetics which may lead to the alleviation or abolition of a major mental handicap, should all individuals with a mental handicap be barred from the opportunity of contributing to this research. This question is especially pertinent if it means that other groups in society have to shoulder the burden of the research.

These principles, taken together, enable the nurse to undertake a very effective ethical review. In reviewing other people's research, however, it is unlikely that the ethics of the proposed study will be addressed quite so explicitly. However, there are a number of ethical expectations that the review should seek to have fulfilled by the study:

1. That an appropriate level of ethical review was gained (not just sought) by the researcher.
2. That appropriate technical and professional support was available to the researcher throughout the study.
3. That in undertaking the research, if the researcher is a nurse, the UKCC Code of Professional Conduct has not been breached.
4. That resources have not been wasted in replicating work in an area that has already been adequately researched, or that because of inadequate preparation an impossible research project has been attempted.

And then there are the six expectations identified by Phillips (1986):

5. That the author(s) duly credit other people's work and ideas.
6. That, as well as reporting the positive findings of the study, the author should indicate the negative and contradictory findings.
7. That the researcher report the limitations of the data and any problems in the study that influence the interpretation of the data.
8. That when interpreting the data and describing the implications of the study the researcher should stick firmly to the facts.
9. That in reporting the results of the study the researcher should present the findings in a scientific manner and avoid sensationalising the results.
10. That the researcher should not pretend that a theoretical base for this study preceded the data collected when it did not.

These ten points provide a framework for a quite thorough ethical review. The final topic covered in this section is what to do when these expectations are not fulfilled. The first point is to check the nature of the report to see whether a fuller account which might fulfil all the expectations is available elsewhere. Next, it is worth getting a second opinion on one's own view about the study. Third, try to contact the researcher to check with him any personal concerns and, if these are justified, to press for subsequent publication to fulfil the expectation. Finally, if the concerns cannot be allayed, then the findings of the study must be evaluated in the full knowledge that it is not ethically sound and that therefore, as a reader, you have good grounds for rejecting the findings of the study.

(f) Evaluating the usefulness of research

The concept of usefulness in research is often difficult to explain. There is one school of thought which argues that all research is useful because, first, even if the results are not applicable at this moment in time, they may well be in the future; and second, even if it turns out that the research findings could not be applied, then the researchers themselves have learnt something from the experience and it has demonstrated for other researchers the futility of pursuing this approach. The reason that the usefulness of research has been an issue in nursing is that concern has been expressed about the allocation and use of resources when research is, or can be, so expensive and the money and nurses' time could be put to so many other uses.

One fundamental weakness in the way that nursing has built up its research-based knowledge is that until recent years the overwhelming proportion of completed projects have been student projects. The vast majority have been in part completion of masters' degrees or at best doctorates in philosophy. This automatically puts constraints on the study, as the student has to choose a study which can be completed in a comparatively short period of time, with limited resources and where the primary judgement on the piece of work will be whether it fits the academic criteria required for completion of such work by a student, rather than its usefulness to the profession and in the delivery of care. For many student researchers, this requires a sense of pragmatism which enables them to apply themselves to their course needs rather than addressing the great questions of nursing.

The root of the problem is twofold: first, the shortage of resources; second, the profession deciding what it is that needs researching. The shortage of resources can itself be considered under two headings.

First, there is the problem of manpower. Getting the number of nurses trained in research to an advanced level has taken time and in all specialisms except general nursing remains a major weakness in nursing research. In the RNMH syllabus, for example, this might have been due to the low priority given to teaching research and in a research-based manner. Brown and Walton (1984), in their study of how the GNC syllabus for RNMH training was taught, barely mentioned the term 'research' let alone how research was taught. The emphasis in basic nurse education and the availability of first degree courses incorporating a basic statutory course have had a major influence upon the generations of researchers. Students in the field of mental handicap nursing have not had the benefit of either of these.

The second resource problem is one of funding and the provision of research centres for nurses to work in. Reliance upon the government for funding has resulted in a methodological straitjacket being applied which has mitigated against the 'softer' types of research. Further, it has taken nearly two decades to find 'homes' for researchers to base themselves in when undertaking research. Failure by the professions to generate resources in terms of manpower and money has worked against the long-term goal of better care for patients and clients through research-based practice. Further, there is a need for senior NHS management to learn that nurse researchers cannot be shackled with traditional management restraints if good-quality research is to be produced when they are unit-based. The cost of a researcher is far greater than their salary. Initially, the resources for them must be costed in. Subsequently, when the findings become known, the whole costing base of the care delivery system might have to be reviewed: but that's a story for another day!

The usefulness of research, therefore, is a nebulous concept. The two important elements that must be considered are applicability to practice and availability of the necessary resources to evaluate the research produced. To know whether the results of a study are usable requires that the nurse knows her own practice well and has a clear knowledge of the goals of care to be achieved. The availability of resources for evaluation remains a major problem, as little or no money is set aside for replication studies, and while the health service has such poor library facilities. Until these two problems are addressed, we will continue to have major problems deciding on the usefulness of research.

(g) Identifying research problems

Treece and Treece (1982) quote Wilson as saying: 'Many scientists owe their greatness not to their skill in solving problems but to their wisdom in choosing them'. The point being made here is that while there are many alternatives worthy of investigation by research, determining which of them is researchable is a very skilled process. The term 'researchable' is itself open to misunderstanding, because it does not refer to a world in which resources are limitless and researchers are skilled in all alternative research approaches and techniques. Rather, it is a judgement based on a realistic assessment of available resources and the refinement of the problem into a researchable question.

Normally, in nursing research, it is a question that needs answering. It is usually distinguished from what is sometimes known as social mathematics. For example, the degree of bed occupancy can be worked out by simply counting patients in beds, once definitions of 'patient' and 'bed' have been agreed. In contrast, the factors resulting in one level of bed occupancy in one district health authority in comparison with another district may well be a perfectly sound research problem. However, crucial to the process is the necessity for the problem to be perceived as a problem. It frequently requires manipulation and refinement. Rarely is the original presentation of the problem the one that is investigated within a research project.

When reviewing research projects, it is important to look closely at the way in which the research problem was determined. Sometimes it can be placed firmly within a clear theoretical framework; often it exists in isolation and has to be dealt with empirically. Sadly, as a profession, we have yet to determine a process for generating and evaluating research problems. We have not learnt to do this systematically and so prioritise our research needs. When reviewing research reports and when considering any nursing practice, it should be a natural part of the nurse's life to make judgements about whether or not some issues are research problems and to begin to promote from a local level the need for them to be addressed.

How to nurse in a research-minded manner

This heading was posed as a question at the beginning of the chapter. It should be clear up to this point that two major areas of concern have been addressed: first, the sort of knowledge required by a nurse to be research-minded; second, an important activity known variously as reviewing or critiquing research. These two elements combined form a substantial chunk of what is known as research-mindedness, and any nurse who acquires these skills, and uses them (the important part), can truly be said to be research-minded. However, a major problem remains, and that is applying the products of this research-mindedness to practice.

This problem is often described as the *research—practice gap*. It is reminiscent of other supposed 'gaps' in nursing—e.g. the education—service divide and the ward sister—nursing officer split. It is said that such separations can be discussed and perhaps accepted. It seems to suggest that nursing is so rich in resources that we do not need to pull together as a team for the benefit of our patients and clients. One would believe that pragmatism and a wish to provide the best possible service, especially in the deprived elements of the service, would be the catalysts to effect a bridging and eventual sealing of the gap. In the world of research, much thought has been devoted to the problem, particularly as nurse researchers have an ethical commitment to the application of their results to the delivery of patient care whenever that is appropriate.

In what is now a much quoted study about the utilisation of research, Ketefian (1975) investigated what '. . . happens to research findings relative to one nursing practice after five or ten years of dissemination in the nursing literature; or stated differently, to determine whether nursing research makes an impact on practice'. The practice in question was temperature taking. Ketefian chose this because of nurses' widespread practice of temperature-taking and because of the direct applicability of the findings—among other reasons. The findings demonstrated a very low level of uptake. Freda Myco (1981), in a study conducted in Northern Ireland, reported that in the groups reviewed—senior tutors, clinical teachers, nursing officers and ward sisters/charge nurses—the majority reported not applying any research results in their practice. These and now many other studies on both sides of the Atlantic demonstrate that a gap exists between the production of research findings which are clinically applicable and their incorporation into practice. It is clear that a number of assumptions exist which need to be actively considered.

Phillips (1986) addresses a number of these, on the basis of the findings of the studies quoted above. First, the assumption that the production of clinical research findings will result automatically and in the natural course of events in improvements in patient care. This she sees as being essentially false, because a nurse, in order to use research, needs to know not only how to evaluate research, but also how to transfer it into practice—in other words, how to bring about change. Second, that the skills for doing research and using research are the same. Phillips argues that while there is substantial overlap in abilities, the research consumer is concerned with application to specific groups and in identified places with known limitations, rather than with the nature and investigation of the research problem. The third false assumption is that the transfer of research findings is feasible for practising nurses. Two factors would facilitate this: first, if role models were available to demonstrate how it was done; second, if it was clear that nurses were not limited in their roles by the institutions they served and therefore were free to change practice. Until good role models are more generally present in the profession and institutions stop constraining staff to deliver care to rigid patterns, this problem will not be resolved.

It appears, therefore, that in order to answer the question of how to nurse in a research-minded manner, a number of steps have to be taken some of which are the personal responsibility of each and every nurse, while other factors should be the concern of the profession as a whole:

1. Acquire an understanding of how research is done and of the issues involved.
2. Develop the ability to evaluate research.
3. The profession should facilitate the change from a procedure-based approach to care to a principled approach.
4. Change in practice should be encouraged and supported.

While these factors might not encompass all elements necessary to effect a change to research-minded care, they are the basis for its development.

Conclusion

This chapter has provided nothing more than a taste of what for some is a lifetime's crusade—the delivery of better patient care through the performance and application of research. While those with advanced knowledge of research may believe that some of the issues here have been oversimplified, others may feel that the subject has been made unnecessarily complex and obscure. Hopefully, a middle path has been trodden. But lest anyone feel that he or she has been left without a guide down that path, two very important parts of the chapter remain: first, there are the full references, to ensure that the researcher can check on the sources quoted; second, there is a limited bibliography for those who wish to read further.

In summary, becoming research-minded as a nurse is a lifetime's challenge. In order to console those facing the challenge, two thoughts should be borne in mind: first, there are others suffering the same frustration; second, and more important, it is the person you are caring for who will benefit from your efforts. That is the real stimulus and reason for becoming research-minded.

References

Brown, J. and Walton, I., *How Nurses Learn: A National Study of the Training of Nurses In Mental Handicap—Final Report*, University of York, Dept. of of Social Policy and Social Work, 1984, DHSS J/R195/124

Irvine, J., Miles, I. and Evans, J. (eds), *Demystifying Social Statistics*, Pluto Press, 1979

Ketefian, S., 'Application of selected nursing research findings into nursing practice', *Nursing Research*, **24**(2), 89−91, 1975

Macleod Clark, J. and Hockey, L., *Research for Nursing: A Guide for the Enquiring Nurse*, HM + M, Aylesbury, 1979

Myco, F., 'The implementation of nursing research related to the nursing profession in Northern Ireland', *Journal of Advanced Nursing*, **6**, 51−58, 1981

Phillips, L. R. F., *A Clinician's Guide to the Critique and Utilisation of Nursing Research*, Appleton-Century-Crofts, 1986

Royal College of Nursing, *Ethics Related to Research in Nursing*, RCN, 1977

Treece, E. W. and Treece, J. W., *Elements of Research in Nursing*, 3rd edn, Mosby, 1982

United Kingdom Central Council for Nursing, Midwives and Health Visitors, *Code of Professional Conduct for the Nurse, Midwife and Health Visitor*, 2nd edn, UKCC, 1984

Further reading

Introductory texts

Cormack, D. F. S. (ed.), *The Research Process in Nursing*, Blackwell Scientific Publications, 1984

Huff, D., *How to Lie with Statistics*, Penguin, 1973

Ligfit, R. J. and Pillemer, D. B., *Summing Up: The Science of Reviewing Research*, Harvard University Press, 1984

Notter, L. E., *Essentials of Nursing Research*, 2nd edn, Springer, 1978

Pritchard, P. and Walker, V. E. (eds), *Royal Marsden Hospital Manual of Clinical Nursing Policies and Practices*, Harper and Row, 1984

Advanced texts

Abdellah, B. U. and Levine, E., *Better Patient Care Through Nursing Research*, 2nd edn, Collier-Macmillan, 1979

Diers, D., *Research in Nursing Practice*, Lippincott, 1979

Open University, *DE304: Research Methods in Education and the Social Sciences*, Open University Press, 1979

Plutchik, R., *Foundations of Experimental Research*, 2nd edn, Harper and Row, 1974

Polit, D. and Hungler, B., *Nursing Research: Principles and Methods*, 2nd edn, Lippincott, 1984

Smith, H. W., *Strategies of Social Research: the Methodological Imagination*, Prentice-Hall, 1975

Other texts of interest

Bond, J. and Bond, S., *Sociology and Health Care: An Introduction for Nurses and Other Health Care Professionals*, Churchill Livingstone, 1986

Field, P. A. and Nokse, J. M., *Nursing Research: The Application of Qualitative Approaches*, Croom Helm, 1985

Hogg, J. and Mittler, P. G. (eds), *Advances in Mental Handicap Research*, Wiley, 1981

Turabian, K. L., *A Manual for Writers of Research Papers, Thesis and Dissertations*, 1st UK edn Heinemann, 1982

Wilson-Barnett, J. (ed.), *Nursing Research: Ten Studies in Patient Care*, Wiley, 1983

International Journal of Nursing Studies, Pergammon Press

Journal of Advanced Nursing, Blackwell Scientific Publications

Recent Advances in Nursing, Churchill Livingstone (a constantly expanding series)

Any publications in the RCN Editorial Series of Monographs (a constantly expanding series)

Chapter 9   Person to person
by Alison Morton-Cooper

Understanding each other

'I am the pen, without me this paper cannot live'.

In one sentence Spike Milligan (Note 1) has managed to convey the power human beings enjoy in communicating with one another. But who invented the pen? the radio? Who first published a newspaper or employed a Town Crier?

Communication is a vast subject which encompasses a wide and complex range of networks, from telecommunications, to the bell which rings in school to herald the end of a lesson, to the multi-million pound computer systems which can send messages across the world at the touch of a button. For the purposes of this chapter the concept of communication has been refined to communications between two very important groups: mentally handicapped people and the professionals who work with them.

It could be said that wherever we live in the world, on the remotest island or in the most crowded city, communicating with other people is essential to our well-being. The human species has always found ways of communicating need. Neandertal Man (Note 2) instinctively rooted for food, established and protected his territory, found a 'mate', nurtured children and sought to protect them from harm.

In many parts of the world men and women still struggle against the old enemies of starvation, natural disasters and military conflict. In a highly developed Westernised society such as Britain's, poverty and social division are more likely to be communicated by interested pressure groups, local politicians and a wide range of broadcast and published media. Public awareness of the challenges faced by mentally handicapped people's move from institutional to community-based care has largely been raised by a powerful television lobby, assisted by carers or families whose questions and worries were not receiving sufficient attention close to home.

On a very personal level, the skills required to communicate well are probably partly learned and partly instinctive. A tiny baby discovers that crying will attract the attention of his mother, but there are certain other skills he acquires as a toddler which succeed in bringing him exactly what he wants, be it a favourite toy, a cuddle or a chocolate biscuit! 'What do you say?' intones Mother. 'Say thank you to Granny for the lovely present.' Good manners become essential prerequisites to a skilful vocabulary.

Sensory communication—what we see, hear, feel, taste and touch—affects the choices we make every day of our lives. It helps us to decide whether to put on a coat before leaving home in the morning or to take an umbrella; whether we turn out a light before we go to sleep or wear matching socks.

Exercise 1

Consider the following statements:

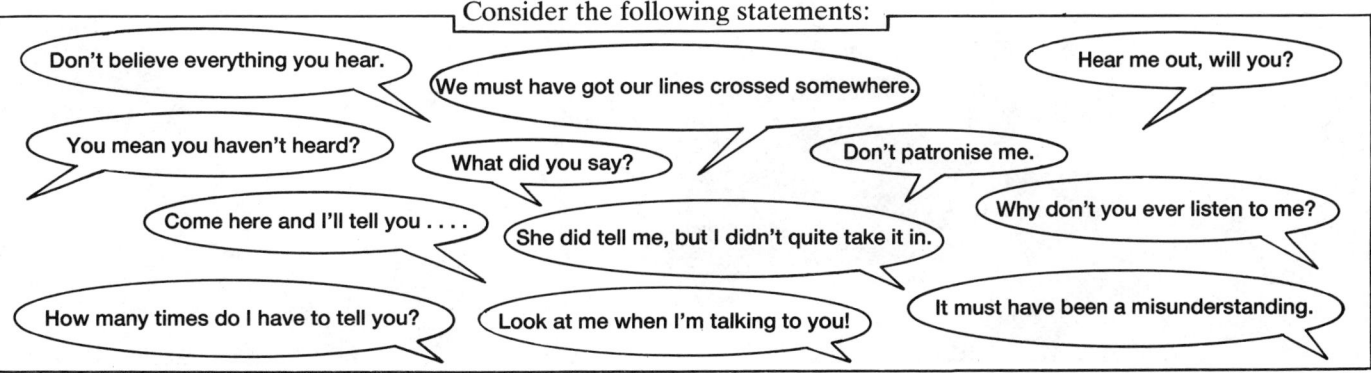

How many times have you heard or used these words? These phrases are a good example of faulty or inconsiderate communication. Poor communication can seriously affect our relationships with people for good or ill. It can make us feel rejected, undervalued; make us suspicious or wary of other people; leave us feeling bewildered, left out, angry and confused. Some statements are more aggressive than others. Can you think of situations where the above words may be used?

As a class exercise, split into groups of three or four and see whether you can put together a short 'role play' using the above phrases. Try to base these on personal experience and improvise as much as possible, so that you are able to express your feelings sincerely.

If one of your group takes the role of a mentally handicapped person, try to assess afterwards the impression he or she gave of that person. What was the result of the exercise? Did the argument become heated? Did feelings of frustration or helplessness emerge, or was the grievance handled diplomatically and sympathetically by the carer and brought to a satisfactory conclusion?

Ineffective communication can render people inefficient, cloud their minds to the really important issues involved, build up unnecessary tensions in relationships, and generally affect personal and corporate morale. Given that a person with a mental handicap may already be limited in speech, movement or hearing, it is easy to see why dependence on carers develops when attempting to sift through information and make proper sense of it.

Sorting through a mass of often complex and conflicting information—i.e. interpreting messages—is a relatively sophisticated process. For example, you have just been told that:

- The food is bad.
- The cook is ill.
- The shops are closed.
- The bus has broken down.
- The bus fare has gone up.
- The bus is full.

These are all very straightforward and commonplace items of information, few of which would present us with any real difficulty in 'coping'. Imagine, however, that for the first time in your adult life you are invited out for a meal by a friend, and you are attempting to put into practice some of those new 'skills' you have learned in hospital or other similar institution. You are waiting for your friend at the bus stop and he is late in arriving. The bus comes. Do you board the bus, even though your friend has not appeared? Have you remembered to allow enough money for the bus fare? How friendly and approachable is the bus driver and where is the ticket machine? Once safely aboard, you decide that your friend will meet you at the café. Ten minutes later, however, the bus begins to make strange noises and stops, and the driver gets out of his seat and leaves the bus. What do you do now? Another passenger, seeing that you are concerned, tells you that he thinks the bus has broken down. Is this

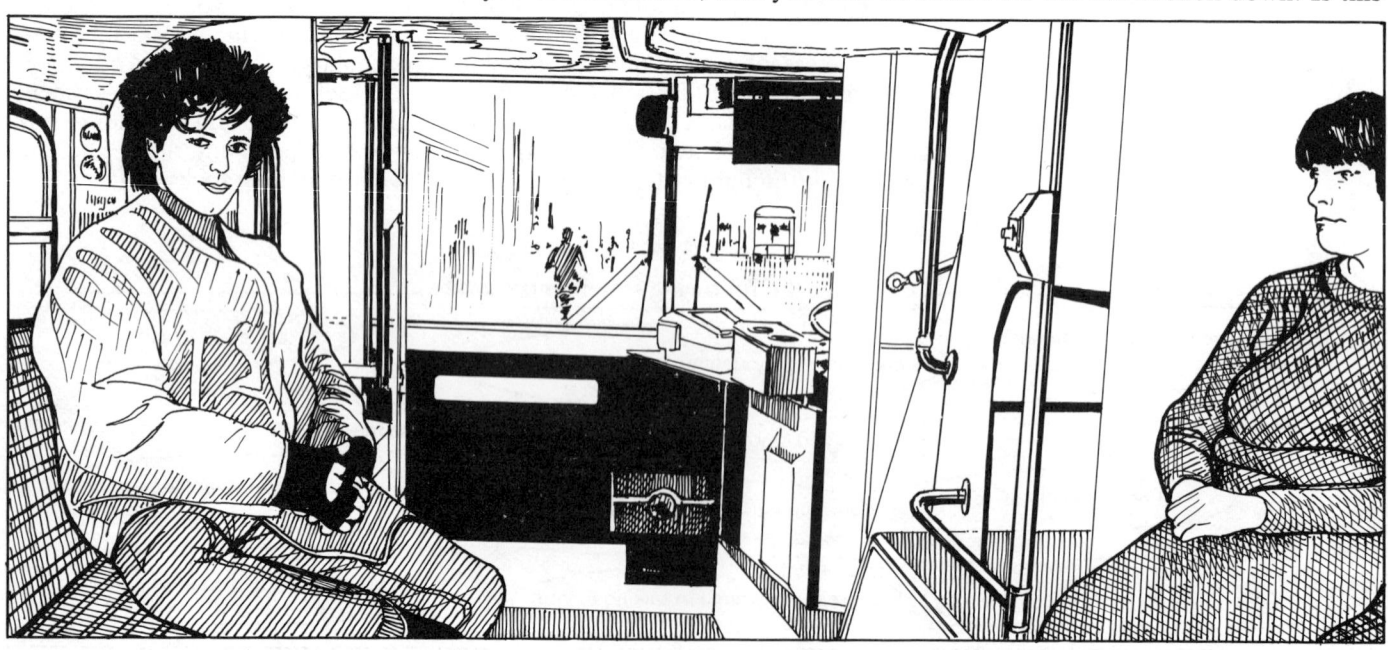

information helpful? What do you do in response to this information? Possible thought processes are:

- What is 'broken down'?
- Why has it broken down?
- Who is going to mend it?
- When is the next bus?
- Will my friend worry about me?
- Now I'll miss my dinner.
- I shall never get home.
- Where shall I catch another bus?
- I shall walk to the café.
- I will leave the bus.

Your success in coping with this catastrophe depends a great deal on the helpfulness of others, such as the bus driver or conductor, other passengers, the bus inspector, and so on. One obvious reaction of someone who has in the past been highly dependent on others is: 'I ask someone to take me home' or 'I shall tell a policeman'.

The points made here may seem terribly obvious. Even so, they require detailed and considered examination, as they illustrate very clearly and simply how important basic communication skills are to a person with limited personal experience of social interaction.

Acquiring new skills

As a nursing student you will be introduced to new concepts of communication as they are relevant to your delivery of nursing care. These skills might include:

- Nurse-to-nurse reporting skills.
- Writing skills.
- Listening skills.
- Verbal skills.
- The ability to reason critically and modify your interventions or behaviour accordingly.
- Teaching skills.
- Counselling skills. (These may or may not constitute a part of your early nurse education. This depends largely on the interests of your tutors and the attitudes of professional colleagues.)
- Intuitive skills (an ability to sense and be aware of undercurrents and unexpressed feelings or needs).
- Touching skills (the ability to convey empathy and understanding within mutually acceptable boundaries).

Most of us appreciate that the ability to speak directly to each other can be inhibited by the following factors: limited speech, a limited vocabulary, shyness, mood (if a person is tired, irritable, affected by alcohol or other mood-altering drug); if a person is startled or frightened, intimidated, cannot see the person he is talking to, or has difficulty in hearing. Similarly, excitement, poor memory or a sense of being ridiculed can also stand in the way of effective and useful conversation.

Awareness of these inhibitions and a willingness to overcome them or make allowances for them can help when working with one another to improve proper lines of communication. Less easy to deal with, and symptomatic of a situation where inhibition presents real difficulties, is the question of *physical* contact. This is often considered a very important part of *non-verbal* communication.

Sexuality and mental handicap

Experience has shown (Note 3) that problems perceived by nursing staff employed in residential care settings for the mentally handicapped are sometimes based on the lack of formal and evaluated sex education for residents.

An interesting debate exists as to whether the teenager with a mental handicap experiences similar 'growing-up pains' to the 'normal' teenager and whether he therefore requires guidance and information on what is happening to his body and how to cope with these physical and emotional changes.

The British are well known for their inhibitions regarding sexuality and intimate matters. With the possible exceptions of Arab and Asian cultures, we would probably be hard pressed to find a culture with more euphemisms for basic bodily functions than the embarrassed British! Certain unwritten ground rules and a mountain of statute books contain fitting testimonies to this supposition.

Few things engender strong public feeling more than the suggestion that sexual habits be discussed openly. Codes of behaviour exist to create boundaries as to what constitutes socially acceptable physical contact between individuals. Add to that the belief that one party is vulnerable (for example, a child, an immature person, or one who is disabled) and these become at once much stricter and carry much more serious consequences for anyone who 'breaks the rules'.

Nowhere is the subject of sex more contentious than in a residential care setting where young mentally handicapped people may become sexually precocious, and where care staff may in certain situations find themselves attracted to someone in his or her care.

It is vital that such contentious issues be addressed carefully and sensitively before they happen. Most parents have difficulty in discussing sex with their young; therefore it is no shame to admit that the subject presents problems in a residential or custodial setting. Care must be taken to ensure that the mentally handicapped person's natural sexual feelings are not dismissed or treated in a derisory way.

Staff must be encouraged to come to terms with their own feelings about this. A properly planned and implemented programme of sex education for clients (and staff!) must be undertaken, and proper guidelines set so that everyone can gain some experience in coping with the client's natural curiosity about his body and his emotions, including sexual arousal.

Exercise 2

Decide which of the following situations constitutes acceptable 'touching'. Discuss these with colleagues and tutors and see how opinions vary.

1. Three-year-old children holding hands in a nursery game.
2. Mother and daughter walk arm in arm on a shopping trip.
3. An 18-year-old female nursing student holds the hand of an 18-year-old mentally handicapped youth while on an outing from the hospital to the local park.
4. A 40-year-old charge nurse hugs an elderly mentally handicapped lady when he wishes her a 'Happy Birthday'.
5. A 40-year-old male nurse holds the hand of a 38-year-old female client while on a 'ward' outing to the pictures.
6. A community mental handicap nurse hugs his 18-year-old girl client in her parents' living room. She has found a job and he wishes to congratulate her.
7. The nurse in a charge of a short-stay hostel walks up to a resident and taps him on the shoulder to tell him that he's late for supper.

At what point does touching cease to be acceptable and friendly and start to constitute suggestive or threatening behaviour? How easily explanations could be given for each of these actions and how easy it would be to misconstrue them!

Well-established systems already exist to allow for communication of need between the carer and his client, such as Makaton sign language. It is much more difficult to find a reliable way of passing and interpreting physical messages without causing people to become anxious or lose confidence when confronted with more complex sexual 'overtones'. Throughout this book it has been made clear that personal attitudes have a tremendous influence on the way we behave as nurses. Space does not permit a lengthy treatise on many of the other skills mentioned above, but it is enough, for the moment, that you are aware of their existence and the need to develop them as you advance in your chosen work.

As a final exercise, you may like to put those 'avenues' of communication open to you as a student to the test, and see whether you can find satisfactory answers to the following questions. Remember always that the power to ask questions, and keep asking them, is part of your raison d'être as a student. It is probably one of the most powerful communication skills you will ever use!

- Are there any laws regarding sexual intercourse and the mentally handicapped person? If so, what are they and what relevance do they have to the nurse–client relationship?
- Who is responsible for educating the young people in your care about their sexuality?
- Is there a recognised formal programme of sex education or is it taught piecemeal or even not at all?
- What happens when a mentally handicapped boy or girl approaches puberty? What is the policy in your care setting regarding the support and guidance required by this young person and his or her parents?
- Are such matters discussed openly between carers and clients, and if not, why not?

Notes

1. Spike Milligan, a poem from 'Open Heart University', Penguin, 1983.
2. Neandertal man was a type of primitive man living in Europe in late Palaeolithic times. The name is derived from Neandertal, a valley in West Germany where anthropological discoveries of his existence were made in 1857.
3. The number of qualified mental handicap nurses appearing before the Professional Conduct Committee of the UK Central Council for Nursing, Midwifery and Health Visiting on a charge of professional misconduct involving a mentally handicapped person or persons (1986).

Further reading

Craft, M. and Craft, A., *Sex and the Mentally Handicapped*, Routledge and Kegan Paul, 1986

Morton-Cooper, A., *The Nursing Student's Handbook*, Chapter 6 'Developing Good Communication Skills', Blackwell Scientific Publications, 1985

Chapter 10   The spiritual dimension
by Peter Birchenall

Spiritual care and normalisation

Any discussion which centres around spirituality, worship and mental handicap must have as its central core the concepts of normalisation and free will. 'Normalisation', in particular, has become an accepted part of nurse education programmes in recent years, but even so, there are conflicting opinions within the profession as to its precise meaning.

For the purposes of this chapter, normalisation will be defined as: 'being in a position to pursue those activities which together form part of normal existence, this to include all things spiritual and temporal'. Free will is a logical extension of normalisation, and should be seen in the context of representing an individual's right to self-determination. By reflecting upon these two major aspects of human existence, we say that to deny anyone the right of access to those things which promote spiritual growth is to fly in the face of the main principles embodied within normalisation, which includes the upholding of an individual's right to worship, according to his faith.

The interested reader may, at this stage, wish to reflect on the work of Nirje. He is one of the original writers on normalisation (Nirje, 1976), and talks of people having opportunities to experience the established activities of daily living through interaction with those elements of society which form the very fabric of normal life. His general principles of normalisation have universal appeal, and can easily be applied to all creeds and cultures.

He underlines the importance of those activities that contribute to a normal rhythm of the day, the week and the year. These activities encompass each and every aspect of human existence which for many people quite naturally embraces a spiritual dimension.

Most religions have special occasions, special times, special actions and rituals which give them structure and order. Such activities are linked with happenings which bring together particular thoughts and emotions. For example, occasions such as Christmas, Passover, or one of the Islamic festivals such as Mawli an-Nabi (the festival of the Prophet's birthday), provide opportunities for family and friends to share in significant happenings within their particular religion. Additionally there are spiritual milestones such as Baptism and Confirmation.

(a) The growth of spiritual awareness

Birchenall and Birchenall (1976) suggest that mildly mentally handicapped people should be able to follow the general meanings within a normal family-style church service. They go on to say that such people are in a position to take a degree of meaning from the Gospel of Christ and are thus able to grown in faith. This point of view is supported in the literature, where it is suggested that even the more profoundly handicapped may understand far more than they are given credit for. This leads into the question of how far does having a normal intellectual level equate with the establishment of faith?

For many people, who are not mentally handicapped, the experience of discovering God is often an unexpected happening and then expressed in a way which is particular to them. Individual differences will determine how people demonstrate their inner feelings to others, especially as spiritual growth is a long-term process requiring some degree of rational thought.

> **Food for thought**
> Reflect on your own attitudes towards the relationship between intelligence and spiritual belief.

(b) Spirituality and interpersonal relationships

A growing spiritual awareness can be strengthened through receiving guidance and support from friends who themselves are going through the same experience. The realisation of this leads to a conclusion of just how important other people are when the neophyte Christian is finding his feet. As McMurray (1961) points out, we are wrong to believe that the individual human unit is a person; it is at least *two people*, because we are only persons in relation to one another. In simple terms, spiritual awareness can only become reality through personal interaction.

Spirituality in a religious context may be equated with the growth and maturity of the human spirit. Developing an understanding and appreciation of the environment within which one lives, and facing up to life with all that it brings, often calls for strength of purpose and the help of others. People certainly gain additional strength from their religious beliefs and affiliation to a particular church. Such strength often results from an understanding of the value of prayer, and also from peer group support.

This then raises serious questions concerning the spiritual well-being of the profoundly mentally handicapped individual. It also brings us to the interface of normality and personhood, which depends greatly upon an individual's ability to reason intelligently and integrate with his peer group. Intelligent reasoning enables us to accommodate the demands of life through skills necessary for the activities of daily living. Intelligence enables us to make rational decisions when faced with several options, and it is this ability which eventually brings many people to accept their faith. Without the ability to decide what is acceptable to us and what is not, we would remain in a state of confusion, unable to make sense of our surroundings or develop any sort of spiritual insight. Intelligence moderates our actions towards others, and through this we come to understand the other person's position, without necessarily accepting it.

> **Food for thought**
>
> Consider how such a belief in a link between ability and faith disables the person in your care. Once again, question your own values and how these influence the level at which you facilitate the spiritual awareness and growth of those in your care.

(c) Spiritual growth and severe mental handicap

To become a fully integrated person within the community, it is necessary to pass through the difficult barrier of self-appraisal and the general acceptance of others. It is probably accurate to say that most people with moderate-to-severe mental handicap would find this difficult, and in some cases highly unlikely. The criterion of dependence/independence can be used to highlight the problems faced by a small but significant section of the population. By some cruel quirk of nature or accident at birth, people are denied the very substance of a rational productive existence and are confined to a life of almost total dependence on others for even their most basic needs. Such an existence gives no real opportunity for inner spiritual growth or the nourishment of the human spirit, both of which are important when coming to terms with the meaning of Christianity. It gives no real opportunity to experience the joy of seeking a lifetime relationship with the Almighty, because the concepts involved are complicated and require a level of awareness which profoundly mentally handicapped people do not have.

There is, however, another side to this argument and perhaps we should be asking ourselves questions of a much simpler nature. For example:

- Do you feel that by asking whether mentally handicapped people can reach God we are doubting God's ability to reach them?
- Does rationality of thought really equate with spiritual growth?
- Do religious organisations encourage the participation of the profoundly handicapped in the sacraments, or are they conveniently forgotten?

By taking the Anglican faith as an example, perhaps all that people with mental handicap require is for the Church to open the way and positively encourage parents to seek Confirmation for their offspring.

A case study revealing a parent's growth of awareness

Offered here is a true case study revealed during an open discussion attended by the author.

The father of a 22-year-old profoundly physically and mentally handicapped woman described his daughter as 'pretty well helpless'. She does nothing for herself, but attends a local day centre as a way of providing her with a change of scenery, as well as giving some means of relief to her parents. There was some evidence of development up to the age of 12 years, but little appears to have happened since that time, and even when she reached 12, her cognitive level was little more than would be expected of a 6-month-old child. With regard to perception, she certainly recognises certain people and responds non-verbally to conversation and music; she also responds to her environment. This is verified by certain reactions observed when she is exposed to differing situations. Her formal verbal skills are nil: except for a few odd noises, she makes no attempt to make recognisable sounds. Non-verbally she can transmit emotion through facial expression: glowering; teeth grinding; and smiling. Physically she is quadriplegic and suffers from hiatus hernia, but, apart from occasional digestive upsets, she is assessed by her father as a happy, loving and easygoing young woman.

The family are regular churchgoers and she receives a blessing from the priest when the Eucharist is celebrated. It had never really occurred to her parents that Confirmation was a possibility, and this threw into stark relief the notion of 'denial of access' to the sacraments. Indeed, the denial of access to many other aspects of normal living features strongly in the lives of people with profound mental and physical handicap. It transpired from the discussion that such denial is often not intended as a deliberate act of discrimination; rather it is a failure to appreciate that even the most severely handicapped person may well respond to external stimuli in the most surprising way.

Food for thought

Consider the notion of 'denial of access' and apply it to the wider aspects of a mentally handicapped person's life.

(d) Present developments

An Anglican priest was also present at the discussion mentioned above and he told of a group of mentally handicapped people and their carers who visited his church for the purpose of partaking in Communion. Despite some problems with motor control when holding the chalice, and a healthy appetite for the pleasant-tasting wine, the handicapped people displayed a natural and simple grasp of the faith, which seemed to emanate from the faith of those who cared for them.

The sacrament is tactile and received in an uncomplicated manner which is highly suited to people with profound handicap. Perhaps it is time to put aside some of the arguments against Confirmation of profoundly mentally handicapped people and accept that Communion without Confirmation may well be acceptable at the discretion of the priest. Such a way forward is seen by Bradford (1985) as having distinct advantages in long-stay hospitals. He says:

'(a) it would enable a sacramental experience to be made available to all mentally handicapped patients who so desired—the majority of whom are reported to find this a particularly meaningful action;
(b) it would avoid any unfortunate discrimination between the confirmed and the unconfirmed;
(c) it would discount any question of "mass confirmation".'

In some cases, Communion without Confirmation may lead towards individuals wishing to undergo some form of training with a view to becoming full communicating members of the church. Bradford suggests a form of preparation involving simple devotional techniques. He proposes art workshops with a faith orientation; mime as a vehicle for faith expression; sharing in selected outside church contacts; and engaging in Christian music therapy.

Food for thought

Consider the nurse's role when preparing people with mental handicap for Confirmation. Explore the contribution of various activities—e.g. art, mime and music—when designing a workshop.

The role of the Church

This seems a relevant point at which to debate the role of the Church as an organisation, and to investigate its integral structures and the part they could play in supporting people with a mental handicap. The Church as a community within itself exists to serve the wider community. It is, as Canon John Tiller (1983) wrote, 'A community of interest, though not merely as a leisure time activity; one of place, though not limited to sanctuary; one of relationship, though not exclusive to any stranger'.

The Christian Church is an enigma; it may appear to the layman as a place where the faithful go to worship each Sunday, or to be visited on those three well-known occasions of baptism, marriage and funeral. To others it represents the very foundation of human existence, and they, in return for the spiritual support it offers, give a resilience and vitality to the meaning of Christianity. Through reflecting on Tiller's description of the Church it becomes clear that as a 'community of interest' it is quite capable of embracing each and every corner of humanity.

It offers an opportunity for individuals to become part of a corporate body, each member being an integral link of the worshipping community. There is no discrimination: the Church is international and culturally diverse; it thrives on its capacity of acceptance based on the fundamental truth that Christ died for us. It is therefore not exclusive to any elite group, thereby placing an onus on local congregations to welcome the most profoundly handicapped person into the Church.

Food for thought

Do you care for residents who express a wish to go to church? How would you facilitate this, especially if different faiths are involved?

Structurally, the Church offers several useful avenues of acceptance; play-groups, Sunday schools, house groups, family services, children's workshops, and social activities are each representative of the network of Christian activity to be found in most parishes. Bayley (1984) places great emphasis on the importance of acceptance where families containing a mentally handicapped member are concerned. He takes as his starting point the view that a mentally handicapped person and his family almost certainly will have experienced some form of rejection. This leaves feelings of vulnerability and an acute sensitivity to further rejection.

My recent experience of a local church youth fellowship entertaining a group of profoundly mentally handicapped adolescents from a long-stay hospital is worth recounting. The regular members displayed a willingness to accept their guests for what they were; everyone enjoyed the party, and games and refreshments were shared in a convivial atmosphere.

Similarly, playgroups and workshops seem to have little difficulty in assimilating mentally handicapped children into their ranks. Children and young adults have few hang-ups about accepting people with mental handicap. The problem seems to lie with adults accepting people with mental handicap as adults themselves! Bailey shares this view and says of 'acceptance':

'However, it is important to recognise that if the handicapped person's behaviour is a bit bizarre, like rocking to and fro and grunting, especially if he is an adult, it may be more difficult. This may indeed test the extent to which a congregation has really accepted the handicapped person and his family.'

Such are the difficulties in this respect that clearly some flexibility in the way that services are arranged may be necessary to accommodate the mentally handicapped person. Bailey suggests an accentuation of non-verbal activity such as gestures, movement, and colourful objects and music, and he calls on other parishioners to act as good role models for the handicapped person. There is every likelihood that positive responses would be forthcoming from everyone concerned—it just requires a little patience and understanding.

(a) Preparation for community living

There is a growing need for the Church to realise the problems which exist for individuals who leave long-stay hospital accommodation for life in a small community-centred dwelling. Many face major readjustment problems and, despite the philosophy of normalisation, will require supervision and support for extended periods of time. A number of districts have set up community mental handicap teams to attend to some of the difficulties, but other districts have yet to do so. Despite the reluctance of some local authorities to recognise the need for multi-specialist teams in the area of mental handicap, it is the Government's policy to phase out large hospitals in favour of community care facilities. The Church as a whole must be in a position to offer pastoral support wherever necessary. Parish priests would welcome any information regarding new parishioners and, better still, the inclusion of a priest on the local community team would be an admirable step in the right direction. Birchenall and Birchenall say in support of this:

> 'The Church is a valuable community resource, guided by the very principles of humanity necessary to welcome strangers, especially those with some form of disability. The cost of going to church is set by the individual to a large extent . . . there is a central focus of belonging that is classless and demands no intelligence tests or hidden skills. As a focus in the community the Church is unrivalled.'

Care staff must accept some responsibility for ensuring that residents' spiritual needs are given identical priority with other facets of community life. During the resident's settling-in period a tour of the local facilities should include a visit to the parish church and an introduction to the vicar. Such an action would ensure that contact is made between resident and clergy which may prove to be highly beneficial. Spiritual care is equally as important as physical and psychological care—it must not be neglected.

Food for thought

When preparing residents for community living, would it be a good idea to familiarise them with local churches and the times of services?

The role of the nurse in spiritual care

An examination of the nursing role in the context of spiritual care must begin with a realisation that not all nurses are believers, and some may find it difficult to facilitate any kind of religious endeavour. This places greater responsibility on those nurses who *do* believe, and they have a specific role in raising the awareness of others involved in care, which includes parents and relatives, to the realisation that, wherever possible, opportunities should exist for the enhancement of spiritual growth. Community nurses may also discover parents of mentally handicapped children who attend church without fully involving their offspring in church activities, such as garden fêtes, parish outings or the act of worship itself. This, again, could provide grounds for gentle discussion regarding the possibility of involving the child in some aspect of church life.

The emerging role of the mental handicap nurse brings into sharp focus the new responsibilities which are rapidly becoming part of her day-to-day work. In recent years a dramatic move away from the clinical model has meant a shift in emphasis towards a model of care based on helping a person towards independence, either wholly or in part. There are new skills to be acquired, particularly those related to effective communication, counselling and teaching. Nursing skills in the modern age are practised within a social network of community care. Part of the knowledge base for successful practice in the community is a thorough understanding of family and institutional dynamics, and how these affect the life-style of individuals. Ayer and Alaszewski (1984) refer to phenomena called kinship ties which, they say, determine an individual's social status and identity; without such ties an individual becomes a 'non-person'.

There are a substantial number of residents living in long-stay hospitals and community-based residences who have no kin. They are dependent on those around them for family support and love. Nurses are in the unique position of providing this essential prerequisite to a normal life-style, and in so doing should always remember that the Church is itself one large family. Every member is a brother or sister to all others, and there is no such thing as a 'non-person' in the eyes of God.

Conclusion

This chapter has addressed itself to some of the main issues facing nurses when called upon to assist those in their care towards spiritual fulfilment. There can be little doubt that with the increase in community care, and a growing awareness within religious organisations of the part they can play in providing a community resource for people with mental handicap, nurses will require to understand more about the spiritual dimension of care. In the past it has received polite but cursory attention within nurse education. This must change, especially as powerful voices throughout the profession are rightly insisting upon an holistic approach to care. The spiritual dimension is one major aspect of this approach and cannot be ignored.

> **Food for thought**
>
> 'By accepting the need for spiritual care, one must begin with the premise that man is a creature with a spiritual dimension, his spiritual needs being viewed in relation with other, physical, psychological and social needs.' (McGilloway and Myco, 1985)

Bayley provides us with 'Ten Commandments' for our Relationships with Persons with Handicaps. For the purposes of this discussion, four of the Commandments are particularly useful and these are reproduced below.

> III. I name you My children: therefore, let no one else define My sons and daughters. Call no one 'crippled' or 'disabled'. There are persons; persons WITH disabilities—individuals WITH handicaps.
> IV. Fear not one another: I know the confusion of your embarrassment, your fears, your anxieties. Your brother's handicap, your sister's disability confronts you; you too are vulnerable. You are both in My care. You are one in My sight.
> VIII. Be grateful for the inspiring quality of life within persons with handicaps, which in turn engenders within all of you perseverance, humour, coping abilities, patience and creative victory.
> IX. Recognise in that community you all share there is also frustration, anger and despair, reminding you all of your common frailty and common need for salvation, and calling you to mission, to provide succour and justice for all.

References

Ayer, S. and Alaszewski, A., *Community Care and the Mentally Handicapped*, p. 154, Croom Helm, 1984

Bayley, M., *The Local Church and Mentally Handicapped People*, p. 5, CIO Publishing, London, 1984

Birchenall, P. and Birchenall, M., 'Caring for Mentally Handicapped People: The Community and the Church', *The Professional Nurse*, 1, 148–150, 1986

Bradford, J., *Preparing the Mentally Handicapped for Confirmation*, Church of England Children's Society, 1985

McGilloway, O. and Myco, F. (eds), *Nursing and Spiritual Care*, Lippincott Nursing Series, Harper and Row, 1985

McMurray, J., *Persons in Relation*, Faber and Faber, 1961

Nirje, B., 'The Normalization Principle'. In Kugel, R. B. and Shearer, A. (eds), *Changing Patterns in Residential Services for the Mentally Retarded*, President's Committee on Mental Retardation, Washington DC, 1976

Tiller, J., *A Strategy for the Church's Ministry*, CIO Publishing, London, 1983

Further reading

Buchanan, C., Lloyd, T. and Miller, H., *Anglican Worship Today*, p. 30, Collins, 1980

Webster, A., A review of *The Local Church and Mentally Handicapped People* (Bayley, M., 1984) in *Parent's Voice*, **34**, 24–25, 1984

Useful addresses

Association of Dance Movement Therapy, 99 South Hill Park, London NW3 2SP

Association of Professions for Mentally Handicapped People, Greytree Lodge, Second Avenue, Greytree, Ross-on-Wye, Herefordshire HR9 7EG

British Association of Art Therapy, 13c Northwood Road, London N6 5TL

British Association of Dramatherapists, PO Box 98, Kirbymoorside, York YD6 6EX

British Association of Music Therapy, Harperbury Hospital, Harper Lane, Shenley, Radlett, Herts WD7 9HQ

British Institute of Mental Handicap, Wolverhampton Road, Kidderminster, Worcestershire DY10 3PP

Castle Priory College, Thames Street, Wallingford, Oxon, OX10 0HE

Dramatherapy Consultants, 6 Nelsons Avenue, St Albans, Hertfordshire, AL1 5RY

The Kings Fund Centre, Albert Street, London NW1 7NE

Royal Society for Mentally Handicapped Children and Adults (MENCAP), 123 Golden Lane, London EC1Y 0RT

The Spastics Society, 12 Park Crescent, London W1N 4EQ

Index*

* Page numbers in *italics* refer to figures on those pages.